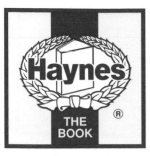

Haynes
THE
BOOK

Weight Loss for Men
Manual

Dr Ian Banks

Cartoons by Jim Campbell

Models Covered
All large sizes, shapes and colours

(5547 - 160)

ABCDE
FGHIJ
KLMNO
PQRST

© Ian Banks 2011

ISBN **978 0 85733 547 0**

British Library Cataloguing in Publication Data
A catalogue record for this book is available from the British Library.

Printed in the USA

Haynes Publishing
Sparkford, Yeovil, Somerset BA22 7JJ, England

Haynes North America, Inc
861 Lawrence Drive, Newbury Park, California 91320, USA

Haynes Publishing Nordiska AB
Box 1504, 751 45 Uppsala, Sweden

HAYNES PUBLISHING: MORE THAN JUST MANUALS

Haynes Publishing Group is the world's market leader in the producing and selling of car and motorcycle repair manuals. Every vehicle manual is based on our experience of the vehicle being stripped down and rebuilt in our workshops. This approach, reflecting care and attention to detail, is an important part of all our publications. We publish many other DIY titles, as well as many books about motor sport, vehicles and transport in general.

Website: www.haynes.co.uk

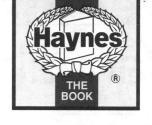

MHF

The Men's Health Forum's mini-manuals contain easy-to-read information covering a wide range of men's health subjects.

The Men's Health Forum's aim is to be an independent and respected promoter of male health, and to tackle the issues and problems affecting the health and well-being of boys and men in England and Wales.

Founded in 1994, The Men's Health Forum is a charity that works with a wide range of individuals and organisations to tackle male health issues. Well established and with an active membership, we work for the development of health services that meet men's needs and help men take more control of their own health and well-being. Our members, partners, staff and trustees bring plenty of experience in health care, media, business and activity.

Men's Health Forum, 32-36 Loman Street, London SE1 0EH

020 7922 7908

Website: www.menshealthforum.org.uk

Website: www.malehealth.co.uk   (for fast, free, independent health information from the Men's Health Forum)

Our registered office is as listed above.

A registered charity (number 1087375). A company limited by guarantee (number 4142349 – England).

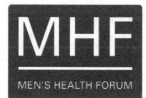

The Author and the Publisher have taken care to ensure that the advice given in this edition is current at the time of publication. The Reader is advised to read and understand the instructions and information material included with all medicines recommended, and to consider carefully the appropriateness of any treatments. The Author and the Publisher will have no liability for adverse results, inappropriate or excessive use of the remedies offered in this book or their level of effectiveness in individual cases. The Author and the Publisher do not intend that this book be used as a substitute for medical advice. Advice from a medical practitioner should always be sought for any symptom or illness.

Contents

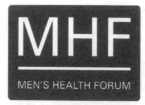

The author, the publisher and the Men's Health Forum would like to thank the following organisations for their contributions to the content, production and distribution of this manual.

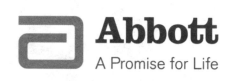

Abbott Laboratories

Abbott Laboratories is a global, broad-based healthcare company devoted to the discovery, development, manufacture and marketing of pharmaceuticals and medical products, including nutritionals, devices and diagnostics.

The central purpose of the company is to develop breakthrough healthcare products that advance patient care for diseases with the greatest unmet need, and improve people's lives.

Abbott Laboratories employs more than 60,000 people and markets its products in more than 130 countries.

In the UK, Abbott employs over 3,000 people, exports products to more than 70 countries worldwide, and makes a significant contribution to the UK balance of payments.

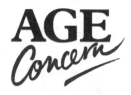

Age Concern

Age Concern campaigns and works for everybody's future. The issues affecting older people today concern us all. We work all over the country making more of life for older people and are supported by a vibrant network of volunteers.

Nationally, we take a lead role in campaigning, parliamentary work, policy analysis, research, specialist information and advice provision, and a wide range of training.

Innovative programmes provide healthier lifestyles and provide older people with opportunities to give the experience of a lifetime back to their communities.

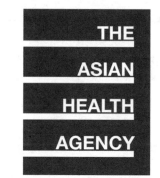

The Asian Health Agency

The Asian Health Agency is a registered charity specialising in the provision of direct and holistic health & social care services and capacity building support services primarily to Asian and other BME communities as well as research, training, consultancy support to statutory and voluntary sectors. particularly in the field of developing culturally appropriate services and anti-discriminatory practices.

TAHA manages over 15 projects centred around London and Slough regions providing a range of services including respite and day care for older people, carers' support services, advice information & advocacy, mental health and counselling, services for people with disabilities, health education and health promotion, capacity building programmes for voluntary and community sectors, parenting programmes for Asian and refugee communities, seminars and conferences and other support services.

TAHA also specialises in developing effective collaborations and programmes to tackle institutional racism and inequality and ensure that mainstream agencies, professional practice and services remain responsive relevant and accountable to Asian and other BME communities.

For further information contact: Balraj Purewal by telephone: 020 8577 9747
email: admincore@taha.org.uk
www.taha.org.uk

ASSOCIATION FOR THE STUDY OF OBESITY

The Association for the Study of Obesity (ASO)

The Association for the Study of Obesity (ASO) is a multi-disciplinary group of professionals concerned with the prevention and treatment of obesity and related diseases. Founded in 1967 the ASO is affiliated to the European and International Associations for the Study of Obesity.

The aims of the ASO are to:
- Promote professional awareness of obesity and its impact on health.

- Educate and disseminate recent research on the causes, consequences, treatment, and prevention of obesity.
- Prioritise obesity and provide opinion leadership in the UK.

We hold regular scientific meetings and a series of training courses for practitioners at all levels. We provide a media information service on obesity and contribute to policy-related discussions and debate.

For further information please see our website (www.aso.org.uk) or contact Ms C Hawkins, Administrative Officer, Association for the Study of Obesity (chris@aso.ndo.co.uk).

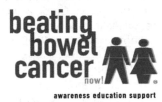

Beating Bowel Cancer

Beating Bowel Cancer is a national charity working to raise awareness of symptoms, promote early diagnosis and encourage open access to treatment choice for those affected by bowel cancer. Through our work we aim to help save lives from this common cancer, the UK's second biggest killer cancer.

We provide information, education and support to bowel cancer patients, their families, the general public and the medical profession.

Beating Bowel Cancer relies almost entirely on the hard work of dedicated fundraisers throughout the country, and we also organise numerous fundraising events and campaigns throughout the year.

For further information, free bowel cancer booklets, or to support our work, contact us on 020 8892 5256 or email info@beatingbowelcancer.org

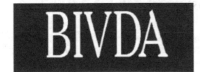

The British In Vitro Diagnostics Association (BIVDA)

The British In Vitro Diagnostics Association (BIVDA) is the national trade association for the In Vitro Diagnostics (IVD) industry. This is the industry which develops and manufactures tests used largely in hospital laboratories to measure substances in blood and other biological samples but also includes self-testing such as pregnancy kits.

BIVDA aims to increase awareness of the difference diagnostics can make to success of the healthcare in both clinical and financial terms. Increased use of diagnostics can save money long term by diagnosing or ruling out disease. Diagnostics are also used to monitor treatment, screen for disease and to ensure the safety of blood used in transfusion.

Contact BIVDA at 1 Queen Anne's Gate, London, SW1H 9BT, United Kingdom (website: www.bivda.co.uk).

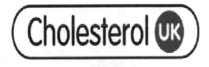

BT Group plc

BT Group is one of Europe's leading providers of communications services and solutions. Its principal activities include local, national and international telecommunications services, higher-value broadband and internet products and services, and IT solutions.

In the UK, BT serves over 20 million business and residential customers with more than 29 million exchange lines, as well as providing network services to other licensed operators.

Further information can be found at: www.btplc.com/Thegroup/Companyprof ile/InvestorInsight.pdf.

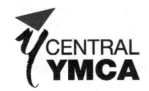

Central YMCA

Central YMCA is the World's founding YMCA, established in 1844 and today internationally renowned for educational programmes within the field of health and fitness. Through three of its operations; Central YMCA Qualifications, the Central YMCA Club and its subsidiary charity YMCA Fitness Industry Training, the organisation is at the forefront of developments and delivery in exercise related training and qualifications for fitness and health care professionals. Central YMCA is actively working at many levels; from gym member to student fitness professional, local authority to Sector Skills Council and with government. The charity's expertise is increasingly being called upon by organisations outside the fitness industry, as exercise is now recognised as an important and effective intervention in the prevention and treatment of many medical conditions.

For more information visit www.ymcaclub.co.uk, www.cyq.org.uk or www.ymcafit.org.uk.

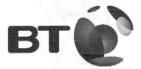

A joint initiative of H•E•A•R•T UK
and the British Cardiac Patients Association

Cholesterol UK

Cholesterol UK is an active advocacy coalition of two charities, HEART UK and the British Cardiac Patients Association (BCPA).

Cholesterol UK campaigns for policy change to achieve:
- A greater focus on high cholesterol levels as a serious risk factor for heart disease and stroke in the wider population.
- Greater awareness of ways to decrease cholesterol levels through diet and lifestyle changes.
- Increased awareness that unhealthy raised levels of cholesterol can contribute to heart health risk in obesity and diabetes.
- Greater access to heart health check-ups, including cholesterol tests, to motivate individuals to improve their heart health.
- Practical guidelines for healthcare professionals to help individuals adopt healthier diet and lifestyles.

Cholesterol UK
35 Bedford Row
London, WC1R 4JH
Tel: 020 7400 4480
Fax: 020 7400 4481
E-mail: info@cholesteroluk.org.uk
www.cholesteroluk.org.uk

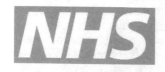

The Department of Health

The Department of Health's activities to improve diet and nutrition and tackling obesity include reducing the consumption of fat, salt, sugar in the diet, as well as increasing physical activity. The 5 a day programme recommends a variety of a least 5 portions of fruit and vegetables a day.

Increasing intake of fruit and vegetables can help you achieve or maintain a healthy weight, as well as help to reduce the risk of coronary heart disease and some cancers.

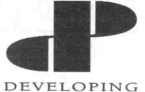

Developing Patient Partnerships (DPP)

Developing Patient Partnerships (formerly Doctor Patient Partnership) is a health education charity working with primary care organisations, employers and the public to make the most of health services and help people manage their health by improving health knowledge and communication. DPP membership includes PCTs, GP surgeries, pharmacists and workplaces across the UK.

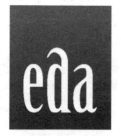

Eating Disorders Association

Eating Disorders Association is a UK wide charity providing information, help and support for anyone affected by or caring for someone affected by an eating disorder, in particular, anorexia nervosa, bulimia nervosa and binge eating disorder.

103 Prince of Wales Road
Norwich
NR1 1DW
Tel: 0845 634 1414
e-mail: helpmail@edauk.com
Minicom: 01603 753 322
Website www.edauk.com
Youthline (Up to 18 years of age)
Tel: 0845 634 7650
e-mail: talkback@edauk.com
txt: 07977 493 345

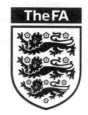

The Football Association

The Football Association is the governing body of football in England, bringing together football's many constituent parts, including 37,500 clubs and millions of players, officials, administrators, managers, coaches and supporters at all levels.

Our role is to promote, develop and regulate the game. That means, in addition to running the men's and women's national sides and a range of national competitions, including The FA Cup, we enforce the laws of the game and promote best practice in a wide range of areas – from financial management to nutrition and fitness.

Perhaps most importantly, it means investing in the long-term future of football – to give everyone the opportunity to enjoy the game. In the last three years, The FA has invested £150 million back in to the game, creating new and improved facilities, training new coaches and supporting schools football.

Football is the national game in England and has enormous potential to improve the nation's health and well-being. Together with our partners in the sport, we are working to harness that potential and encourage as many people as possible to take part, get fit and have fun.

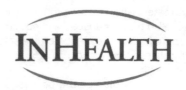

InHealth Group

InHealth Group is a leading provider of healthcare services to the NHS and independent health care sector, having developed proven, expert and marketing-leading clinical managed services that directly support health professionals in the pursuit of outstanding patient care. Through two of its operating divisions, Cardinal InHealth and Lister InHealth it delivers a cohesive and leading edge range of clinical solutions.

Cardinal InHealth is the UK's leading provider of mobile and modular Cardiac Catheterisation services. With over 11 years experience delivering a wide range of cardiac managed solutions, Cardinal InHealth has extended its portfolio to include Myocardial Perfusion Scintigraphy and Digital Mammography.

Lister InHealth is the UK's leading provider of MRI, CT and PET scanning services, carrying out over 220,000 procedures a year. Lister InHealth, like Cardinal InHealth, provides both facilities and staffing on either a short or long term basis, operating fully managed services in either a static or mobile environment.

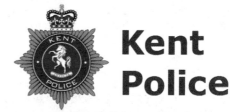

The Kent Police Service

Kent Police delivers policing to 1.6 million people through its 6,000 officers and staff across 20 locations in Kent. We aim to work with partners to create a safe environment for everyone in Kent, where they feel protected by a visible and accessible police service, displaying a sincere commitment to reducing crime and disorder.

We also aim to maintain the integrity, quality and effectiveness of policing services. In order to maintain an effective service, Kent Police recognises the vital need to maintain the health of its workforce and is delighted to support this manual.

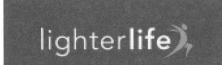

LighterLife

Founded in 1996, LighterLife is a medically monitored weight loss programme for the obese. Using a nutritionally complete Very Low Calorie Diet in conjunction with Cognitive Behavioural Therapy, clients step back from conventional food to enable them to be in ketosis which blunts hunger, whilst the CBT counselling helps them to explore the reasons behind their overeating. In the 'men only' groups, the average weight loss is three stones in nine weeks. There is a Management Programme to help clients maintain their weight loss over the long term. LighterLife is an organisational member of BACP and a member of the British Nutrition Foundation.

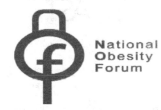

The National Obesity Forum

The National Obesity Forum (NOF) is an independent medical organisation, whose aim is to raise the awareness of obesity as a serious medical condition and to promote best quality management within the NHS. The NOF provides evidence based clinical guidelines for medical management of adult obesity, childhood obesity (in association with the Royal College of Paediatrics and Child Health) and for pharmacotherapy for obesity, which have been widely published and utilised by health authorities within the UK and internationally. It awards the annual 'Award for Excellence in Obesity Management in Primary Care' and has published educational material for all healthcare professionals on paper, CDRom and on our website. There is an

annual NOF conference on the clinical management of obesity. The NOF is a first port of call for professional advice to the media on all obesity related issues. The NOF helped establish the All Party Parliamentary Group on Obesity in 2002, continues to provide professional and secretarial support to the Chairs, Dr Howard Stoate MP and Mr Vernon Coaker MP, facilitating four parliamentary meetings each year, and has provided expert opinion for the National Institute for Clinical Excellence (NICE).

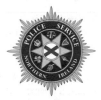

POLICE SERVICE of NORTHERN IRELAND

The Police Service of Northern Ireland

The Police Service of Northern Ireland is committed to making Northern Ireland safer for everyone through professional, progressive, policing. It has a workforce of approximately 9,000 police officers and 3,500 support staff and is one of the largest employers in Northern Ireland. Vital to the success of policing is the health and physical fitness of all our employees, consequently the PSNI Human Resource and Occupational Health strategy recognises the importance of the workplace when tackling health issues. Significant benefits have already been gained by addressing these issues through the provision of a voluntary well person screening programme called 'Health Patrol' for all our staff. We are delighted therefore to be associated with the production of this manual and the undoubted contribution it will make to the health of our staff and the nation as a whole.

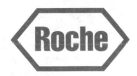

Roche

Roche aims to improve the health, quality of life and well-being of people in the UK through our innovative range of

diagnostic and pharmaceutical products that focus on the needs of individuals.

This breadth of interest enables us to take an integrated approach to healthcare, focusing on the prevention, diagnosis and treatment of disease and the enhancement of well-being.

Part of one of the world's leading healthcare companies, Roche is proud to have been a part of the UK's healthcare environment since 1908. Today we employ around 1,800 people based at two main sites in Welwyn Garden City, Hertfordshire, and Lewes, East Sussex.

For more information, please visit our website at www.rocheuk.com.

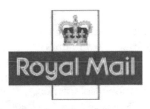

Royal Mail Group

Royal Mail Group plc operates as three well-known and trusted businesses: Royal Mail, Post Office®, and Parcel Force Worldwide, with a turnover of £8 billion.

Royal Mail's 140,000 postmen and women use a fleet of 30,000 vehicles and 33,000 bicycles – and their feet – to collect, sort and deliver 82 million letters each day to the nation's 27 million addresses.

ParcelForce Worldwide's employees operate in a competitive market for express deliveries, and the Post Office® employees run the UK's largest retail chain providing 170 products and services to 28 million customers each week.

As the largest employer of men in the UK, their health is vital to our success, and we are delighted to support this manual.

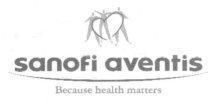

sanofi-aventis

The sanofi-aventis Group is the world's 3rd largest pharmaceutical company, ranking number 1 in Europe. Backed by a world-class R&D organization, sanofi-aventis is developing leading positions in seven major therapeutic areas: cardiovascular disease, thrombosis, oncology, diabetes, central nervous system, internal medicine, vaccines. The sanofi-aventis Group is listed in Paris (EURONEXT : SAN) and in New York (NYSE : SNY).

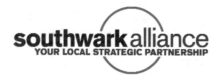

Slim Fast

Slim Fast has been the world's most popular meal replacement weight loss programme for more than 15 years. Its simple structured programme of nutritious meal replacements, satisfying main meals and snacks has been proven to help people lose weight and maintain that weight loss for years. Used with equal enthusiasm by Olympic athletes and housewives, Slim Fast is the perfect weight loss plan for people with less time to prepare food, or who need to follow a diet when they are constantly on the go.

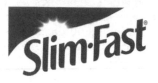

Southwark PCT and Southwark Council

Southwark PCT and Southwark Council are jointly developing, as part of their neighbourhood renewal strategy, an extensive programme to improve the health of men, in particular targeting the most derived neighbourhoods. The Southwark Men's Health Programme provides nurse-led outreach MOTs; referral to indoor activities, such as self-defence, swimming and kick boxing; outdoor pursuits such as gardening, accompanied walks, tennis and organised sports; healthy eating advice, cooking and weight management; confidence building workshops and anger management; and personalised smoking cessation and lifestyle programmes.

For more information, please contact mens.health@southwarkpct.nhs.uk or visit: www.southwarkpct.nhs.uk/menshealth

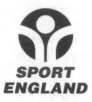

Sport England

Sport England is the strategic lead for Sport in England and invests Lottery and Exchequer funds into sport. Our aim is to encourage people of all ages to start, stay and succeed in sport at every level and make England the most active and successful sporting nation.

Sport England has nine Regional Sports Boards (RSBs), each made up of experts from areas such as business, local government, sport, health and education. The RSBs provide the strategic lead for sport in their regions and distribute investment for grassroots sport. Sport England has invested more than £2bn of Lottery funds into sport across England and more than £300 million from the Exchequer.

To find out more, visit: www.sportengland.org

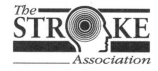

The Stroke Association

The Stroke Association is the only national charity solely concerned with combating stroke in people of all ages. We are doing more to help people affected by stroke by providing stroke patients and their families with support through our community services. These include Dysphasia Support, Family Support, Information Services and Welfare Grants. Campaigning, educating and informing to increase knowledge of stroke at all levels of society. We also act as a voice for everyone affected by stroke. Funding research into prevention, treatment and better methods of Rehabilitation.

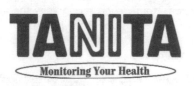

TANITA

Tanita has been a global leader for more than half a century in developing products to help people enjoy a healthier life. In 1992, Tanita developed the world's first stand-on body fat monitor and is now the international market leader in BIA technology led products. Our products are widely used both in the home and professionally by medical and fitness experts.

As part of Tanita's family ethic the company operates a community investment programme regularly contributing to medical research, local charities and working closely with organizations that address health related issues.

For more information on our professional or home use products visit www.tanita.co.uk

The Obesity Awareness & Solutions Trust

The Obesity Awareness & Solutions Trust (TOAST)

The Obesity Awareness & Solutions Trust (TOAST) is a national advocacy charity which is dedicated to encouraging a better understanding of obesity, its causes and practical solutions through stimulating informed debate, developing and delivering training packages about and researching aspects of obesity. Equal opportunities are at the core of all of TOAST's activities and service development is led by needs as identified by the people who use our service, that is people who are overweight as well as carers and professionals. TOAST runs an information desk for the obese, overweight, post obese, compulsive overeaters and for those who work with obesity or the obese. They launched a National Help and Advice Line in March 2005. They are also piloting a number of proactive programmes such as training packages aimed at professionals in all areas including health and education and in Life Management to arm the overweight and obese with the skills to be comfortable with their bodies and manage their weight over an entire lifetime.

Registered charity number: 1088049

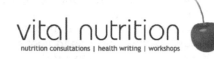

Vital Nutrition

Vital Nutrition is an independent, Belfast based company, offering health workshops for private and corporate clients, one-to-one nutrition consultations for individuals (at Framar Health, Belfast) and health writing for various publications, including local and national newspapers and magazines.

To contact Vital Nutrition, telephone Jane McClenaghan on 0775 969 0701 or email info@vital-nutrition.co.uk.
Vital Nutrition
PO Box 430
Belfast
BT8 7YA
www.vital-nutrition.co.uk

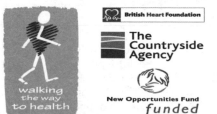

Walking the way to Health

'Walking the way to Health' (WHI) is an initiative of the British Heart Foundation and the Countryside Agency. It benefits from extra funding from the New Opportunities Fund. WHI aims to improve the health and fitness of more than one million people, especially those who do little exercise or who live in areas of poor health, by getting them walking more in their own communities.

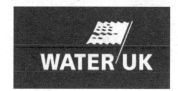

Water UK

Water UK is the industry association that represents all UK water and wastewater service suppliers at national and European level. We provide a positive framework for the water industry to engage with government, regulators, stakeholder organisations and the public. We actively seek to develop policy and improve understanding in areas that involve the industry, its customers and stakeholders.
www.waterforhealth.org.uk

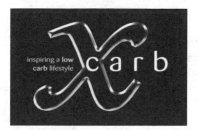

Xcarb

Xcarb is an exciting offer of low carb products that has been created to tackle the current obesity crisis head on. In doing so, it has gained the support of leading health experts, the medical profession, and also the National Obesity Forum.

Based in the UK, Xcarb is dedicated to supporting the 21% male population now classed as obese and the quoted three million people in the UK currently watching their carb intake. Its main objective, however, is to help make a real difference and at the same time make life easier for those watching their waistline.

The complete Xcarb range offers real food for real people covering breakfast, lunch, dinner and snacking on the go. It gives people the opportunity to lose weight by eating real foods without having to compromise on their favourites such as bangers and mash, cereal or even pasta with sauce.

The products – that not only taste superb, but are also nutritionally balanced and healthy – are available in supermarkets throughout the UK. Those wishing to find out more can visit www.xcarb.co.uk.

Acknowledgments

Charities, organisations, government bodies and industry are all credited in this manual but individual writers, without whom this HGV Man Manual would be yet another 'diet book', deserve grateful acknowledgment. In no particular order:

David Haslam
Veronica Aldridge
Louise Diss
Martin Breach
Lyndel Costain
Steve Boorman
Paul Lichfield
Steve Deacon
Mark Greener
Susan Jebb
Alan Hardy
Angie Anderson

Anthony Leeds
Ike Odina
Balraj Qadir
Chris Hawkins
Gordon Youngman
Jane McClenaghan
Jim Pollard
Mary Barrington-Moor
Matthew Maycock
Meryl Johnson
Syed Abidi
Pam Prentice
Paul Grassby
Penny Whitecross
Peter Baker
David Wilkins
Samantha Harding
Steve Bloomfield
Andy Beswick
Tara McDowel
Tom Hain

Veronica Aldridge
Ric Coggins
Tracy Burg
Pamela Taylor

Special thanks to Matthew Minter, Ian Barnes and Jim Campbell, who brought to life a very difficult subject. Simon Gregory read the manuscript and gave his expert opinion. The Department of Health was instrumental in producing this manual and recognising the need for information directed towards men themselves.

Dedication

This book is dedicated to all the organisations and individuals whose contributions made it possible. Whilst many hands make light work, too many cooks spoil the waistline.

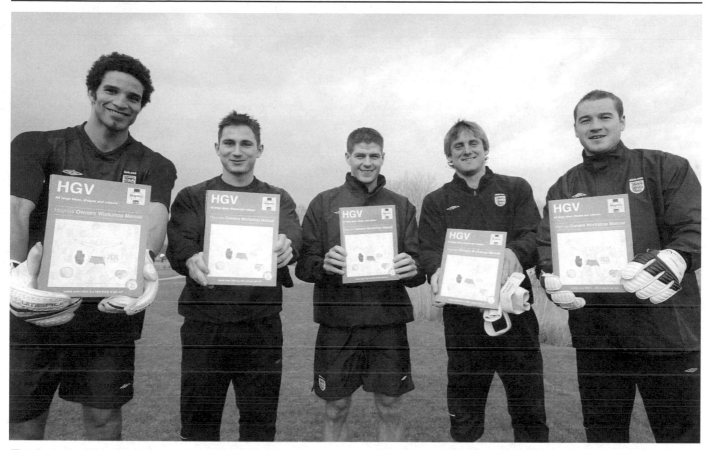

Thanks to the FA for their encouragement and assistance, not least in setting up this photo for us with members of the England squad. From left to right: David James, Frank Lampard, Steven Gerrard, Robert Green, Paul Robinson.

Photo courtesy of The FA

Introduction

Make no mistake, this HGV Man Manual is not another pontificating, finger-pointing bit of heavy goods. It is more than just a book about men and weight. It is fun, functional and totally fat free. It is also designed for men so forget the leotards. This manual will arouse your innermost desires, get your juices going, and reach places no other manual could reach before: your girth.

Not convinced by the weight loss argument? Consider a 2005 report in the British Medical Journal called *'Obese men can regain sexual function by losing weight and exercising'*. Luckily the title of the article gets the message across, because the text is pretty heavy going (*"Interventions focused on modifiable health behaviours may represent a safe strategy to improve erectile function and reduce cardiovascular risk..."*) but basically it confirms that erectile dysfunction is not only reversible, it may not require drugs such as Viagra.

Neither is it simply a diet book - goodness knows the bookshop shelves are creaking under their combined weight. Instead there is a 'History of Gluttony' which makes a lot of us feel better already. 'Eat yourself slim', not all food will bust your belt. Even the FA gets in there with tips on diet and fitness for sportsmen. In fact, just about everything you might want to mentally feast on about weight and wisdom is in these pages.

What you won't find is patronising pap to put you off living. Read on to lighten the load. Keep on Truckin.

Ian Banks

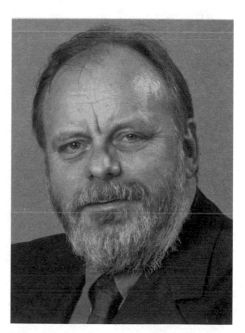

Chapter 1
Right fuel?

Contents

1 Lifestyles costing truckers their health

1 A groundbreaking study carried out in Sefton has revealed that lorry drivers' health is being put at risk by a combination of junk food, smoking and lack of exercise.

2 Truckers using Seaforth Docks told researchers they knew their lifestyles were a problem but said their daily routine gave them little chance of getting any healthier.

3 The study was part of the 'Tommy the Trucker' initiative devised by the local NHS to help reduce 'health inequalities', where specific groups are shown to have poorer health than the population as a whole.

4 It concludes that lorry drivers' lifestyles put them at higher risk of chronic illness such as heart disease, diabetes and cancer.

5 Jo McCullagh of Sefton Health Improvement Support Service explained: "Men in general are less likely to access health services than women, and less likely to receive information about ways to improve their health."

6 "But, compared to other men, we've found that lorry drivers are even more likely to have high fat diets, eat less fruit and vegetables, smoke, take less exercise and be overweight."

7 "It was striking how many of the men we spoke to were worried about the impact it was having on them but,

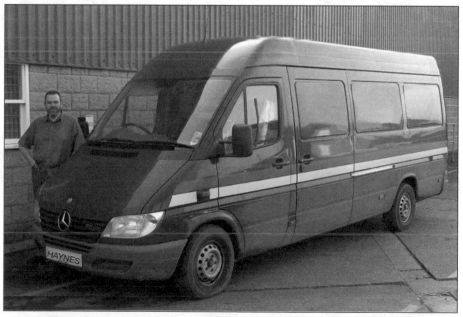

Lorry drivers' lifestyles put them at higher risk of heart disease, diabetes and cancer

because of the nature of the work, didn't know what they could do to look after themselves any better."

8 The team behind the research is now recommending work is done to improve the food on offer to truckers at roadside catering outlets, and that haulage companies provide drivers with cool boxes to store healthy foods like fruit and salad.

9 Their report also suggests installing gyms and shower facilities at major stop-off points so that drivers can enjoy some exercise after spending hours at a time on the road.

10 Gareth Lewis, Men's Health Nurse for South Sefton Primary Care Trust, said: "At the moment, the average trucker's daily routine just doesn't allow for them to lead a healthy lifestyle."

11 "Their working hours make it hard to access health services that are only open from nine to five, and because they are away from home a lot they have little choice as to what they eat or what they do when they arrive at their destination."

12 "The facilities waiting for them when they step out of their cabs have to be more conducive to a healthy lifestyle, or truckers will always face an uphill struggle to be as healthy as the average man in the street."

2 Who ate all the pies!?

DEVELOPING
PATIENT
PARTNERSHIPS

From 'Working Lunches report' (DPP: Developing Patient Partnerships, Sept 2004)

1 Research found that a quarter of men (25%) regularly miss lunch at work, with 32% of manual workers such as factory workers and labourers skipping lunch. According to the research, people are tending to replace lunch time meals with 'grazing' on naughty nibbles which are often high in fat and sugar such as fizzy drinks, crisps and pies.

2 According to the research snacking habits vary depending on where you live…

3 Northerners are the biggest crisp eaters with almost half (43%) saying that they snack on them. Apparently the further north you go the healthier you get

as Scots claim to be the least likely to snack on crisps and a whopping 70% of them reach for the fruit bowl for the healthy snack option.

4 When it comes to pies Northerners come on top again with 1 in 4 of the population reaching for a pie to snack on whilst just 19% of their neighbours in the Midlands would pick a pie for a snack.

5 Sugar seems to have us all stuffed though, as fizzy drinks, cakes and pastries are loved almost the same throughout the land with 1 in 3 (34%) of us plumping for pastries or cakes, and more than a quarter (27%) going for the fizz (and we're not talking pints).

6 Sadly, when it comes to healthy options, over a quarter (27%) of manual workers find healthier snacks too expensive. Amongst all respondents, cost appears to be the main reason stopping people from buying healthier snacks with a quarter of people (26%) saying that they are too expensive and 12% of men finding them boring.

7 But there are many ways to eat healthier snacks and they don't need to cost a bomb. Here are some suggestions on how to liven up your lunch box without having to watch your waistline:

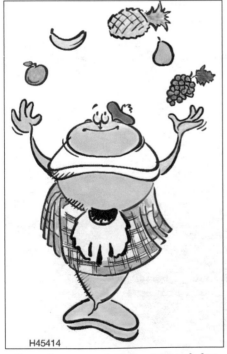

Seventy per cent of Scots reach for the healthy fruit snack option

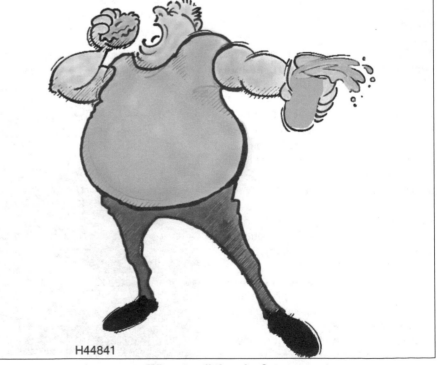

Who ate all the pies?

Less Healthy Snacks	Sat fat	kcals	Healthier Snacks	Sat fat	kcals
1 Slice battenburg cake (50g)	2.5g	185	1 Bagel (70g)	0.7g	188
1 Chocolate bar (60g)	10.7g	317	1 Scone (50g)	1.7g	158
1 Packet crisps (40g)	3.7g	218	1 Currant bun (60g)	1.3g	186
1 Danish pastry (110g)	6.2g	411	1 Slice toast (24g)	-	64
1 Sausage roll (60g)	8.0g	286	1 Crumpet (40g)	-	80
1 Doughnut (80g)	3.4g	318	1 Piece of fruit (80g)	-	20-30
1 Chocolate biscuit (30g)	5.0g	157	1 Box raisins (25g)	-	68
			1 Pkt raisins & peanuts (10g)	1.8g	174
			1 Slice malt loaf (35g)	0.1g	94

Did you know?

- Obese men are 33% more likely to die from cancer than men of healthy weight.
- Two out of every five men in the UK have high blood pressure.
- A man who is two stone overweight is twice as likely to have a heart attack as a man of healthy weight.
- 30 000 deaths a year are directly attributable to obesity – a person dies every 17.5 minutes of an obesity related illness.

- It is predicted that 34% of men and 38% of women will be obese in 2025 and 50% of the population will be overweight.
- 800 000 prescriptions of obesity drugs cost £36M annually.
- Men with a waist circumference of 37 inches have increased health risks, with a waist circumference of over 40 inches they have substantial health risks.
- 40% of advertising on children's TV is for food; 70% is for high energy density food high in salt & fat.

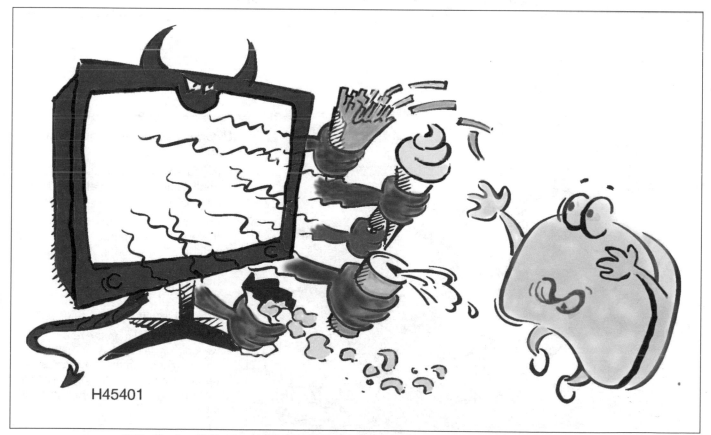

H45401

40% of advertising on children's TV is for food; 70% is for food high in salt and fat

3 Quotable quotes

"Start with the achievable and build on success – anything is better than nothing."   Professor Ken Fox

"The most important thing about motivation is goal setting. You should always have a goal."   Francie Larrieu Smith

"The mechanics of industry is easy. The real engine is the people: Their motivation and direction."   Ken Gilbert

"You are what you think. You are what you go for. You are what you do!"   Bob Richards

"Motivation is what gets you started. Habit is what keeps you going."   Unknown

"Motivation is like food for the brain. You cannot get enough in one sitting. It needs continual and regular top ups."   Peter Davies

"No one does anything from a single motive."   Samuel Taylor Coleridge

"What we see depends mainly on what we look for."   Sir John Lubbock

"In the middle of difficulty lies opportunity."   Albert Einstein

"The mind is the limit. As long as the mind can envision the fact that you can do something, you can do it, as long as you believe 100%."   Arnold Schwarzenegger

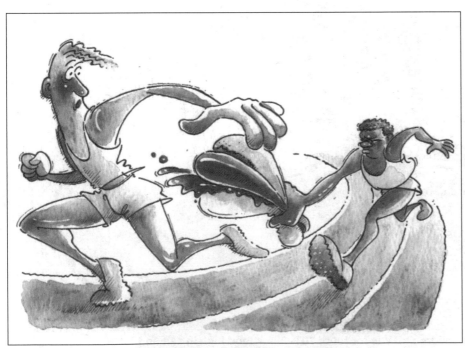

Food eaten whilst on the run has no calories

Free calories?

Unfortunately none of the following is true:

- If you eat standing up the calories don't count. This rule also applies on your birthday!!

- Foods used for medicinal or therapeutic purposes don't count. Things like cough sweets, hot chocolate, toast and marmite, soup, boiled eggs and soldiers, beer, curry after a hard week…

- Broken biscuits have no calories.

- Food eaten whilst on the run, standing, walking or driving has no calories – if you are eating on the run calories used up equate to eight hundred per hour for running and this will negate your intake.

4 You are not alone

Regional breakdown of key press release statistics from 'Get Sussed, Get Healthy Family Challenge Campaign' (DPP: Developing Patient Partnerships).

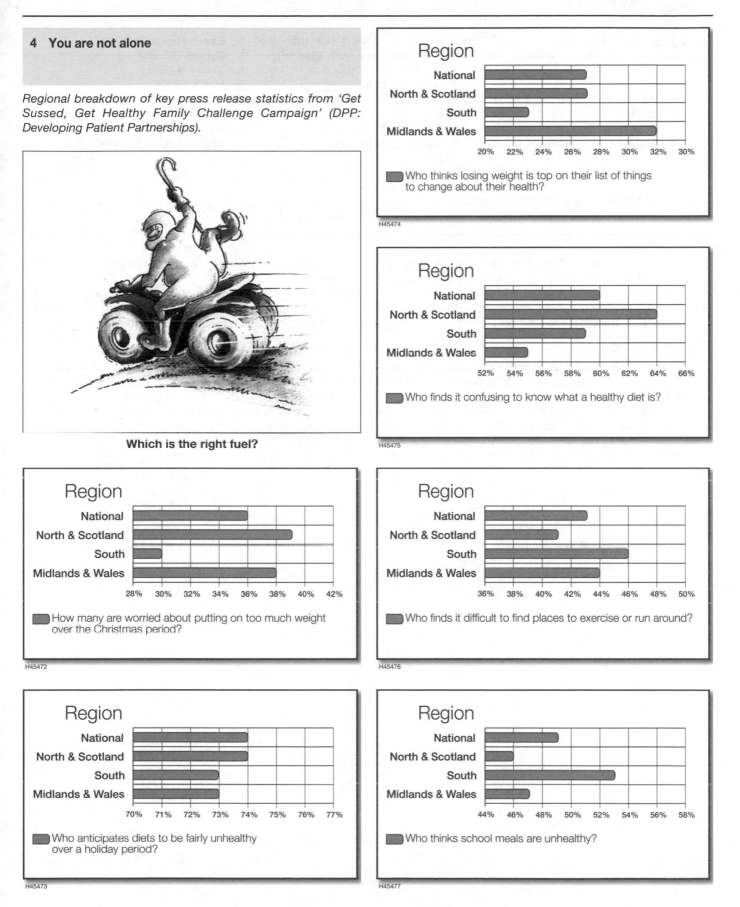

Which is the right fuel?

Region — Who thinks losing weight is top on their list of things to change about their health?
(National, North & Scotland, South, Midlands & Wales; axis 20%–30%) H45474

Region — Who finds it confusing to know what a healthy diet is?
(National, North & Scotland, South, Midlands & Wales; axis 52%–66%) H45475

Region — How many are worried about putting on too much weight over the Christmas period?
(National, North & Scotland, South, Midlands & Wales; axis 28%–42%) H45472

Region — Who finds it difficult to find places to exercise or run around?
(National, North & Scotland, South, Midlands & Wales; axis 36%–50%) H45476

Region — Who anticipates diets to be fairly unhealthy over a holiday period?
(National, North & Scotland, South, Midlands & Wales; axis 70%–77%) H45473

Region — Who thinks school meals are unhealthy?
(National, North & Scotland, South, Midlands & Wales; axis 44%–58%) H45477

5 No fat Frenchmen?

1 Sorry, it's not true. There is a book called French Women Don't Get Fat, but you have to take the title with a (small) pinch of salt. However, plenty of other European nations are fatter than the French, though it's not really clear why.

2 The tubby top ten (from www.malehealth.co.uk):

1. **Greece** (78.6% of blokes are overweight or obese - so much for the Mediterranean diet!)
2. **Germany** (75.4%)
3. **Czech Republic** (73.2%)
4. **Cyprus** (72.6%)
5. **Slovakia** (69%)
6. **Malta** (68%)
7. **Finland** (67.8%)
8. **Slovenia** (66.5%)
9. **Ireland** (66.4%)
10. **England and Wales** (65.4%).

Healthy Cooking Tips from overseas

- Increase the amount of fibre in meals. Include more pulses in meals: for example, try stewed peas/lentils with rice, or yam or sweet potatoes.
- The traditional One Pot Soup (akin to a meat or vegetable casserole) is usually a very healthy option, especially if more peas or pulses are used and less meat.
- If dumplings are prepared, half white flour and half wholemeal or cornmeal should be used.
- Sweet potatoes can be boiled or baked with the skin.
- Reduce fat intake: when and wherever possible cut down on food containing high saturated fats like coconut cream, evaporated milk, etc. Lean meat should be used and remove the skin from chicken.
- Fish, meat and chicken (after being seasoned) should be stewed or baked with little or no fat. Little fat should be used with dishes like 'jollof' rice (recipe with chicken, ham, tomatoes, onion, cabbage and green beans), saltfish (salted cod) and ackee (Caribbean fruit). Plantains (banana-like fruit) can also be baked, rather than fried.
- With soups made with groundnut/peanut or palm oil, allow the soup to cool (after cooking) and then pour off the layer of excess oil.
- Reduce the amount of salt in your diet: gradually cut down on the amount of salt used in preparing food. Many ready-made seasonings contain a fair amount of salt.
- Try using fresh or dried herbs like thyme, coriander, turmeric, paprika, garlic, chilli and black pepper.
- Saltfish, salted mackerel, stockfish (air-cured fish such as cod or haddock) and salted pig-tails are high in salt content and should be soaked overnight in large quantities of water, to remove as much salt as possible, before cooking.
- Try to cut down on salty foods/snacks like bacon/ham, packet/tinned soup, crisps and nuts.
- Fresh fruits are a much better option.

Chapter 2
Losing weight

Contents

1 Are you ready to lose weight for life?

By Dr David Haslam

Choosing your vehicle

1 You may have a multitude of reasons for wanting to lose weight. For example, you may have suddenly noticed your reflection in the mirror and decided to change your appearance, or you may have recently suffered a clinical warning signal such as shortness of breath or frequent tiredness.

2 Whatever your incentive, a weight-loss manoeuvre is usually an extremely sensible option.

3 This is because obesity (defined as having a body mass index (BMI) over 30; see Chapter 5 to work out how to calculate yours), is closely linked to a number of serious, life-threatening diseases. For example, compared to thin people, people who are obese are four times more likely to contract heart disease. They are also more likely to suffer a fatal course of cancer[1].

Fat facts

Being obese increases your chances of developing one or more of these serious medical conditions[2]:

- *Arthritis.*
- *Asthma.*
- *Back pain.*
- *Cancer.*
- *Cirrhosis.*
- *Depression.*
- *Diabetes.*
- *Gallstones.*
- *Gout.*
- *Haemorrhoids.*
- *Heart disease.*
- *Heart failure.*
- *Heartburn.*
- *High blood pressure.*
- *Increased surgical risk.*
- *Infertility.*
- *Stress urinary incontinence.*
- *Varicose veins.*
- *Wound infections.*

Understanding what's under your bonnet

4 If you want to lose weight, it is important that you have realistic expectations.

5 If you feel that you have a lot of weight to lose, it is not a good idea to try to lose it all in one go. A much better idea is to break your overall target into smaller chunks and then aim to lose a small amount at a time. For example, if you would eventually like to lose 25 kg (4 stone), it would be sensible to set an initial target of losing 10 kg (22 lbs).

6 This is an excellent initial target to set yourself because research shows that this amount of weight loss can result in a substantial number of health benefits. Losing 10% of your body weight (eg, 10 kg in a 100 kg man) decreases your chances of dying from an obesity-related cause by around 20%[3].

7 You should also aim to lose weight gradually, so that your metabolism remains high. If you try to lose weight too quickly (ie, by starving yourself), your metabolism may slow right down and go into "starvation mode". This means that your body needs fewer calories to function, so although you have cut down your calorific intake, some calories will still be converted into body fat.

8 A weight reduction of 0.5-1 kg per week is a sensible average rate. To achieve this, you should reduce your calorific intake by 500-600 kcal per day.

9 To lose weight healthily, you should also increase your daily exercise regime, and aim to take 30 minutes of exercise, five days a week.

10 Brisk walking, cycling or swimming are good examples of suitable fat-burning exercises. You should also revert to a low-fat diet.

How to improve your diet

- Do not shop for food when hungry.
- Store healthy foods where you can see them.
- Use smaller plates and utensils.
- Eat more slowly.
- Chew food thoroughly before swallowing.

Your weight-loss journey

11 Your willpower also plays an important part in your weight-loss attempts. If you want to lose weight successfully, you must be mentally ready for the challenge. Put simply, you must be totally dedicated to making the necessary changes to your lifestyle.

12 Making any major change involves six key stages. These stages closely resemble a car journey. Using the list below, at what stage would you currently place yourself?

Leaving the car in the garage (the pre-contemplation stage)

13 At this stage, you have not yet decided that you want to lose any weight.

Getting in the driver's seat (the contemplation stage)

14 At this stage, you have thought about losing weight, but are not yet ready to start.

Starting the engine (the preparation stage)

15 You have decided that you want to lose weight, and are prepared to make the necessary lifestyle changes within the next few weeks. You may already have set a date to start dieting. You may also feel that you need some additional guidance and support to help with your weight loss attempts.

16 Your reasons for wanting to lose weight may be:

- To be able to walk upstairs without panting.
- To look better.
- To be able to wear off-the-peg clothes.
- To lower the strain on your knees.
- To put on shoes and socks more easily.
- To lower your blood pressure.
- To achieve long-term health benefits.

Releasing the handbrake (the action stage)

17 Well done. You have got over the first hurdle and have started to make the lifestyle changes which will help you to lose your excess weight.

Reaching your destination (the maintenance stage)

18 Congratulations, you have reached your target weight. You must now concentrate on maintaining your new reduced weight.

The return journey (the relapse stage)

19 For whatever reason, you have gone back to your old ways of eating too much and not exercising regularly. The weight that you initially lost has started to return. You must find the inner strength to turn your behaviour back around.

20 Whatever stage you find yourself at, your doctor can provide additional help and support. Some of the ways that he can help are listed in the following table.

Stage of your weight-loss journey	How your doctor can help
Pre-contemplation	At this stage, you will not yet have decided to visit your doctor because you have not yet accepted that your weight is a problem. However, if you are visiting your doctor for another ailment, he or she may proactively mention that you should lose some weight.
Contemplation	At this stage, your doctor may be able to help you develop a list of pros and cons associated with your weight loss. For example, you could discuss: • What you will gain from losing weight. • The likely difficulties you will face. • The barriers that are stopping you from losing weight right now.
Preparation	At this stage, your doctor can help you develop a sensible weight loss plan. This could include: • The number of calories to aim for each day. • The types of foods to avoid. • A suitable exercise regime. • A valid start date.
Action	At this stage, your doctor can help you overcome any cravings to ensure that you do not lose sight of your weight-loss goals. In addition, if you are finding it increasingly difficult to stick to your original weight-loss plan, he or she may be able to help you regain your motivation and make the necessary modifications to put you back on track.
Maintenance	At this stage, you are unlikely to need any additional support, as you are managing quite nicely on your own. However, your doctor is always there if needed, and may be able to offer medications to complement your diet and exercise programme.
Relapse	At this stage, you are not likely to visit your doctor as a result of your weight problem because you have lost interest in maintaining your new, reduced weight. However, if you are visiting your doctor for another ailment, he or she will almost certainly ask about your weight, and may try to pursue the triggers that made you revert to your old behaviour. This may help to put you back on track with your weight-loss attempts.

21 One type of weight-loss aid that you can only get from your doctor is medication (eg, sibutramine and orlistat). **22** These two medications can help to boost your weight loss attempts. Both of these medications must be taken alongside a sensible diet and exercise programme, and are only suitable if your BMI is more than 27 and if you have other obesity-related conditions, or if your BMI is greater than 30.

References

[1] Haslam DW. Obesity - the scale of the problem. General Practitioner July 2001; p31-32.
[2] Haslam DW. Time to tackle obesity. Family Medicine February 2000; p25-31.
[3] Colditz GA, Willett WC, Rotnitzky A et al. Weight gain as a risk factor for clinical diabetes mellitus in women. Annals of Internal Medicine 1995; 122: 481-486.

2 Slow down – the lazy man's way to lose weight

1 Men know Diets with a capital D don't work. So how do you build weight-loss into your daily routine?
2 A survey published by Mintel in 2004 claimed that record numbers of men are attempting to lose weight. Apparently one in four of us would like to shift a kilo or two – up from one in six in 1980.

3 Perhaps we've all been inspired by the recent Danish research showing that being overweight lowers your sperm count and makes you less fertile. The University of Southern Denmark found that, compared with men of normal weight, overweight men – defined as men with a body mass index over 25 – had a 24% lower sperm count. (See Chapter 2 to calculate your BMI.)
4 Anyway, regardless of its impact on your fertility, the general tone of the media coverage of the Mintel report was that men trying to lose weight must be a good thing at a time when two-thirds of the male population is overweight or obese. Maybe. But the trouble is that diets don't work. And the whole weight-loss obsession can be very damaging to the self-image. Fortunately, many men already know this. Twice as many men as women told the researchers that they would never diet and only 3% would even consider joining a slimming club.
5 The report found that men tend to want to lose weight for health reasons rather than to get into smaller clothes sizes. As a result we are more likely to cut out the booze or take more exercise than to resort to meal replacements or faddy diets.
6 So what do you do? If you want to lose weight without actually changing what you eat it comes down to two things: slower and fresher.

Go slow

7 To start, don't even think about what you eat. Think about how you eat it. Lots of us stuff our faces in front of the telly hardly noticing what we're shovelling in. No good.
8 Take it easy. Drink some water. Look at your food. Chew it. Savour the flavour. Drink some more water. You'll enjoy your food more and your body will know that it's actually eating. This is vital because when it comes to food your brain's a bit slow. It takes it a good 20 minutes to wise up that your stomach is full. This means that if you've been stuffing yourself, you'll have eaten tons more than you wanted. Good rule of thumb? The first belch. It's dear old mother nature's way of telling you've had enough. (And, of course, like all mothers she does it in the most publicly embarrassing way possible.)

Be a thin couch potato

Don't just sit there. Think thin. Fidget. Sit up violently. Burn more energy by stretching while you yawn. Get up and walk to the TV.

What sorts the bone-idle thin from the most languid obese people? The answer is Neat or non-exercise activity thermogenesis. Neat is more powerful than pumping iron or running on the spot.

Low Neat means obese people sit down on average 150 more minutes each day than even the laziest lean people. Patients with low Neat have a biological need to sit more. The study shows that the calories people burn in their everyday activities – their Neat – are more important in obesity than previously imagined.

The decade-long study required volunteers to wear special underwear that recorded their every movement. They were also given special meals and gave up all unauthorised snacks. Then the scientists tried another regime. They made the thin volunteers consume an extra 1,000 calories a day, and underfed the larger ones by 1,000 calories. Even when they lost weight, the naturally obese moved less, while the naturally thin walked and fidgeted more.
US journal Science Today

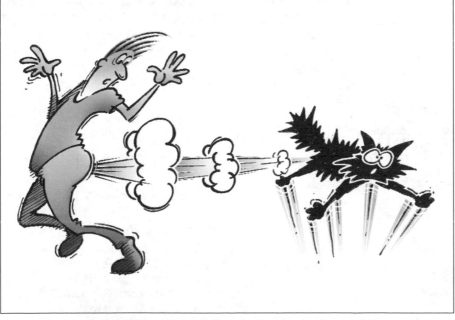

Mother Nature's way of saying you've had enough

Get fresh

9 Once you're eating more slowly you'll taste your food better so the smart next step is to choose the tastiest version of it. Now, I'm no farmer but it's clear that the carrot that tastes most like a carrot will be the one you've pulled out of the ground yourself rather than the one that was picked weeks ago and has since been flown round the world, sliced up, salted, sugared and tinned. The good news is that this fresher version is also the most nutritional version with the most vitamins.

10 So don't change what you eat but choose the least-processed version of it. The more factories and other places your food has been through, the more likely it is to have had sugars, salts and fats added. Avoid ready-meals and convenience pre-packed options. Don't buy a chicken meal, buy a chicken. When it comes to fruit and veg, frozen is better than tinned. Fresh is better than frozen. Organic is better than supermarket.

11 Not that all fresh food is that fresh. If the item has been flown from the other side of the world it's likely to be less fresh than something produced down the road. Check out the country of origin on fruit and veg and buy local.

12 It's hardly brain surgery is it? Baked beans are a good example of the problem with processing. The beans themselves are pretty good for you but in the tins we buy they're pumped up with salt and sugar. Nobody's suggesting you bake your own beans – though you could chose a reduced salt and sugar version – but you see the point.

13 Apart from the reduction in nutrients, processed foods – and fast foods like burgers and fries too by the way – have a high energy density. That means that each mouthful contains a lot of calories. More calories than your body is expecting. Human beings have evolved over thousand of years to guess how much we need to eat by the size of a portion but just an ordinary looking portion of a high-density food can contain double the calories your body expects. If you also have the habit of putting it away like a wolf in a meat factory, you can see how the calories can mount very quickly.

14 Worst of all, you can become dependent on the sweet, salty, fatty tastes because they give you an instant sugar hit. In tests, rats who are used to this sort of food get the shakes when they're deprived of it. Trouble is that the hit soon wears off and you're back starving again. Now, if only you'd eaten more slowly in the first place. Just like mamma used to say.

Get fresher

15 Talking of evolution, you can take that idea a little further and think about what food we've evolved to eat rather than what we actually do eat. Humans have been on Earth for hundreds of thousands of years. In terms of our evolution, the cultivation of crops only began yesterday and the processing of food even more recently.

16 That's why you hear people going on about the raw food diet or the caveman diet. Sure, they're trying to sell diet books but the basic theory is sound. For most of our time on this planet, we would have been eating what we could hunt and what we could gather from the landscape around us. That means a diet of mainly fruit, nuts, vegetables and meat. Not that the meat would be much like today's meat. The meat on a hunted animal is different to the flab on a factory-farmed one that has never seen daylight and never walked more than a yard or two. Lean meat, free-range, organic or game gets a little nearer to what you're after.

17 This is not say you shouldn't eat cereals but that you should try to get the version that's closest to nature. That means whole grain or wild rice. Fresh, wholemeal bread rather than factory white. If you're having trouble eating the government's recommended five portions of fruit and vegetable a day, you'll find it a lot easier if you replace one serving of cereals, bread, pasta or rice with one of vegetables.

18 But sorry, as usual, chips don't count.
19 Why not? Well, since potatoes are pretty disgusting raw (most of their plant relatives are poisonous), we didn't start eating them in quantities until we learned to cook food. Again this happened relatively recently. There's that and the 50g of fat in a portion of fries!

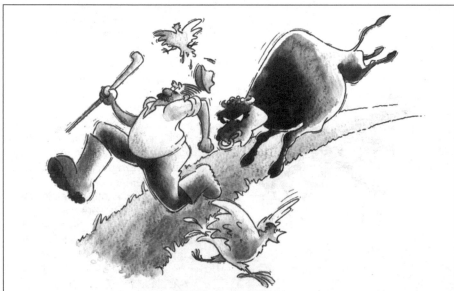

The MOT and servicing that you give your body keeps it running to its optimum

---

3 Goal setting

The Obesity Awareness & Solutions Trust

What is in a thought?

1 The MOT and servicing that you give your car or bike keeps it:
- *Running to its optimum.*
- *Stops it from breaking down.*
- *Keeps it performing well.*
- *Ensures safety.*

2 You will probably spend time, skill, effort, thought and energy looking after your car because you want it to be reliable, efficient and to perform well. You value your machine and your motivation will be to keep it in peak condition (or working at the very least.)

3 When you go to fill up with fuel do you ever put petrol instead of diesel in the fuel tank or visa versa? Unlikely because you think about what fuel your machine needs to keep it working well. It is something that you have done many times and seems automatic to go to the right pump. If you put the wrong fuel in the consequences would be undesirable: the engine would seize up, the machinery would not work and you would end up spending time and money in getting it fixed. Most likely you are also motivated to think about how you treat your vehicle so that it works properly and doesn't conk out.

4 Although MOT and servicing bring with them some trepidation and a set of negative thought patterns about possible failure, for most of us it is also recognised as inevitable and necessary.

5 Do you spend as much time looking after yourself, thinking about what fuel you need to perform well and how best to recharge your batteries as you do on your vehicle?

6 Do you service and MOT your body and mind and consider what will keep you mentally and physically in peak condition? Or even what will keep you functioning well enough so that you can live life the way you want to?

7 Good intentions are often sabotaged by our own 'demons'. Think of all the times that you have been determined to do something like: go to the gym, take the dog for a walk, mow the lawn, walk to work, and take the stairs not the lift. Then the little voice on your shoulder persuades you that: "you'll to the gym and mow the lawn next week, take the dog for a walk/walk to work when it isn't raining and run up the stairs when you have more time." The demons always seem so rational and offer us the easy option.

8 The truth is that what we say to ourselves really does count. Our thoughts affect our feelings and how we feel effects the way that we act; it is the things that we say to ourselves that affect us.

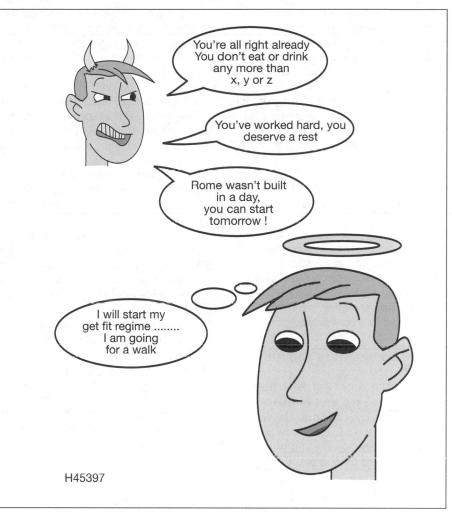

Good intentions are often sabotaged by our own 'demons'

9 As a result, actions are more likely to include withdrawing from people and avoiding new situations, or perhaps acting on our hostility with sarcasm or blaming.

10 Believe it or not, these negative thoughts serve a purpose. If you are anxious about trying something new and your own thoughts say, "I can't do that! I'm a stupid fool to even think of it! " – you are likely to listen, not give it a try, and, sure enough, your anxiety is relieved. The critical voice protects you in a backward kind of way from fear of failure and rejection. Negative thinking may become automatic – ingrained in your self-image and you end up living your life that way.

11 Positive, encouraging interactions during childhood go a long way toward promoting positive self-talk when we are adults. But if that was not the case when you were growing up, it doesn't mean you can't work to develop positive self-talk now.

12 Counter your negative self talk with something more reasoned. It is not always helpful to try to turn a negative thought into a positive one.

13 When you find that demon telling you things like, "I will never get the job…" "I'll never get the weight off…"

14 Ask yourself:
- *Where is the evidence for this?*
- *Is this always true?*
- *Am I looking at the whole picture?*
- *Am I being objective?*

15 Make your decisions based on logical discussion with yourself rather than allowing them to be a *fait accompli*.

16 Remind yourself of some of the successes that you have had in life and remember how good you felt when you achieved them. Did they involve a lot of work along the way that you could easily have talked yourself out of? Sometimes it is not until you feel the pleasure of achievement that you can see that your efforts were worthwhile. When it all seems hard work without instant rewards, and a pie and a pint looks more attractive than a brisk walk or an hour at the gym, remember how good you'll feel when you have achieved what you set out to.

17 Looking after yourself, giving yourself a good service and MOT, and doing the work that you need to do to get you running well, is like that. There will be times that you wonder what you are doing it for. Other times that your demons try to convince you that something else or some other direction would be a better one. Knowing how powerful your thoughts are will give you another tool for your kit bag.

Do you know where you are going?

18 What is it that you think that you want? Are you the sort of person who looks with envy at the BMW your neighbour has and plans how you are going to get one, or are you more likely to look at it and be content with the fact

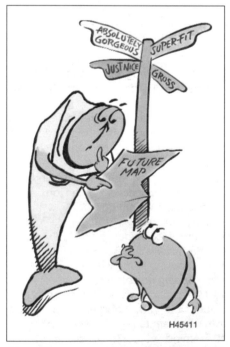

Planning a route and making sure that you know where you are going are useful

that your car is well maintained and reliable?. What do you want for your body, the super model, the perfect body or just one that works well that is well maintained and reliable?

19 When you go on a journey what are some of the things that you need to do before setting off? Planning a route and making sure that you know where you are going are useful. You might look at the map or use a route master. If you are going on holiday you may need to book in advance where you are going to stay and you will either need to save up the money or pay for it later.

20 Life is like that too it takes planning to look after yourself and to know what direction you need to go in but often we take our bodies for granted and forget to plan what we need to keep ourselves in good condition.

21 It is easy to take on board too many calories for a variety of reasons and we don't spend them because we are not active enough to use up the calories that we are eating. We end up in the red and our overdraft of excess calories will be turned into fat. Excess fat will clog up your arteries and put you at high risk of:
• *Heart attack.*
• *Stroke.*
• *Cancer.*
• *Diabetes.*
• *High blood pressure.*
• *Joint problems.*
• *Breathing difficulties.*

22 Is this what you want? Is this what you have but you want to do something about it?

23 In order to plan what you want for yourself and your body you need to know what you want. You need to work out where you are going to be able to know when you have reached your destination. You need to be clear about what you are trying to achieve.

The most important thing about motivation is goal setting

24 Consider these questions:
• *What are your life time goals?*
• *What are your goals for the next three to five years?*
• *What are your goals for this year?*
• *What are the things you need to do in order to accomplish this year's goals?*

25 Now list the things you will do this week, and the things you will do today

that relate to your goals for this year. To this list then add anything else that you want to accomplish during the day or week.

26 You now have a 'to do' list!

27 Ask yourself which of these activities you really enjoy doing. Which do you find hard slog? Which do you avoid doing at all? How many of the things that are hard slog relate to your life time goals? If you find that you are not achieving things that you want to it may be because you are not able to see what the longer term rewards for you will be.

28 Think about the consequences of achieving these goals, and the consequences of not.

29 Some consequences are pleasurable and others are avoidance techniques. The consequences of avoiding something can be very motivating for escape and reinforcing the belief that by avoiding the situation you have protected yourself from:
• *Criticism.*
• *Failure.*

30 And feeding into the, "I knew it would be better not to… apply for the job/join the gym/cycle to work/etc".

31 Pleasurable ones are more helpful for building positive behaviours.

32 Consequences can be immediate or delayed. Consequences serve as more effective motivators if they are immediate. This is why it is easier to eat a pie from the garage, which gives instant gratification, than make a healthier option at home which will take time to prepare and time to see the positive results of looking and feeling healthier.

Immediate
• *Satiate hunger.*
• *Save time.*

Delayed
• *Eat healthily.*
• *Look after myself.*
• *Feel good.*

33 Take some time to work out what keeps you ticking and make sure that you put yourself in the driving seat when it comes to determining what direction your life takes.

34 Remember the most powerful person in your life is you and you can achieve your goals in 1st or 5th gear depending on the speed that you decide to go.

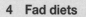

4 Fad diets

Peanut Butter Diet

This diet allows helpings of 6 tablespoons of peanut butter per day, combined with a recommended 45 minutes of exercise per day. The total daily calorie intake on the diet is 1500 calories per day for women and 2200 calories per day for men but, because of the peanut butter content, a slightly higher percentage of calories are derived from fats than on traditional diets.

Advantages

The peanut butter diet combines sensible eating and an exercise program, with regular helpings of a popular comfort-food. Evidence suggests that it actually does successfully deliver slow and steady weight loss, although the weight loss might be a bit faster without the peanut butter.

Disadvantages

This diet may contain nuts!

Conclusion

Sounds a bit nutty, but it is at least an improvement on the doughnut and apple pie diet.

Cabbage Soup Diet

The Cabbage Soup Diet is a 7-day rapid weight loss program, that combines frequent helpings of cabbage soup with portions of fruit, vegetables and grains.

Advantages

A diet that includes home-made soup and other fresh ingredients is likely to be quite nutritious and healthy.

Disadvantages

Even if you start by absolutely loving cabbage soup you will hate it by the end of the week. Any diet plan will be more successful if it is varied, interesting and very tasty.

Conclusion

And the forecast is: it is going to be windy, very windy.

Raw Foods Diet

The Raw Foods Diet recommends eating mainly uncooked vegetarian food. This is a diet high in fruits and vegetables, seeds and nuts; and low in starch.

Advantages

Many foods that can be eaten raw are high in vitamins and nutrients.

Disadvantages

A diet composed exclusively of uncooked foods will not be balanced, easily tolerated, or healthy in the long term, but will at least save time cooking.

Conclusion

Probably best not to eat pork chops on this diet.

Cider Vinegar Diet

According to some, cider vinegar has fat-burning qualities and works to speed up metabolism. The diet involves taking several spoonfuls of cider vinegar with every meal.

Advantages

You can eat whatever else you like.

Disadvantages

The vinegar will taste so awful that you may be tempted to think twice before eating.

Conclusion

Vinegar is good for fish and chips, not losing weight.

Negative Calorie Diet

The Negative Calorie Diet claims that digesting some foods burns more calories than they contain, and that eating other foods actually speeds up your metabolism. In addition it claims that simple breathing exercises can 'turn your body into a fat burning machine'.

Advantages

A diet that is high in fruit and vegetables will be filling and really healthy, even if they are not actually 'negative' calories.

Disadvantages

If you really want to burn calories then start exercising.

Conclusion

Does this diet really work? Negative.

Caveman Diet

The Caveman Diet recommends a diet high in fruits, berries, nuts, vegetables, fish and meat. These are all foods that humans evolved on over millions of years. Other foods, such as grains (found in bread and pastas), beans, potatoes, dairy products and sugars have only recently appeared in the diet. Because we are not truly adapted to eating these 'new' types of food, it is suggested that they may contribute to health problems such as obesity, cancer or arthritis.

Advantages

A diet that contains plenty of fresh foods, fish and some meat is going to be very healthy.

Disadvantages

Getting eaten by Tyranosaurus Rex on the way to the supermarket.

Conclusion

"Wilma! I'll have the Brontosaurus steak!"

Grapefruit Diet

This diet suggests that grapefruit acts as a magical fat-burning catalyst when eaten with other foods. The diet plan therefore combines a low calorie diet with, you've guessed it, a grapefruit with every meal.

Advantages

Grapefruits, like any other fruit or vegetable, are a healthy food; and any low calorie diet will cause some weight loss, at least in the short term.

Disadvantages

Most individuals on a low calorie diet will give up after days or weeks because of hunger: on this diet you might be lucky to last that long.

Conclusion

You may never want to see, let alone eat, a grapefruit again.

Further information

If you would like to know more, look in the Contacts section at the back of the book, or contact:
Website: www.diet-i.com

Recipes

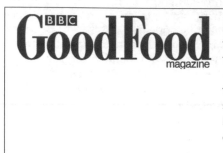

BBC Good Food magazine is a lifesaver for anyone who wants to create easy, tasty, family friendly-meals at home.

With around 100 recipes and meal tips every month, every issue includes simple midweek meals that are ready in half an hour, great ideas for relaxed entertaining, plus inspired dishes from top chefs. Every recipe is foolproof, as they're all thoroughly tested in the Good Food kitchen. In addition, the magazine is packed with food tips, techniques and notes. If you want to enjoy great food at home, you can't go wrong with BBC Good Food.

Published monthly by BBC Worldwide.

Spicy vegetable chapati wraps

Curry can be deceivingly high in fat but our version is packed with flavour and has only 5g of fat per serving.
Takes 20 to 35 minutes.
Serves 4.

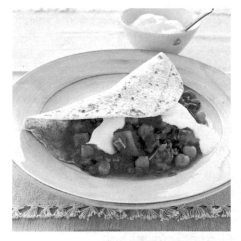

Ingredients

300g/10oz sweet potatoes, peeled and roughly cubed
400g can peeled plum tomatoes
400g can chickpeas, drained
1/2 tsp dried chilli flakes
2 tbsp mild curry paste
100g/4oz baby spinach leaves
2 tbsp chopped fresh coriander
4 plain chapatis (Indian flatbreads)
4 tbsp 0% fat Greek yogurt

1 Tip the sweet potatoes into a large pan of boiling water and cook for 10-12 minutes until tender. Meanwhile, in another pan stir together the tomatoes, chickpeas, chilli flakes and curry paste, then simmer gently for about 5 minutes.
2 Drain the sweet potatoes and tip them into the tomato mixture. Stir in the spinach and cook for a minute or until the leaves have just started to wilt. Stir in the coriander, season to taste and keep warm. Meanwhile, put the grill on to heat.
3 Sprinkle the chapatis with a little water and grill for 20-30 seconds on each side. Put each chapati on a warm plate and spoon the filling evenly between them. Top the mixture with a dollop of yogurt and fold the chapatis in half to serve.

Per serving

289 kcalories
Protein 12g
Carbohydrate 54g
Fat 5g
Saturated fat none
Fibre 5g
Added sugar none
Salt 1.08g

Herbed pork fillet with roast vegetables

Takes 1 hour 30 to 1 hour 45 minutes.
Serves 4.

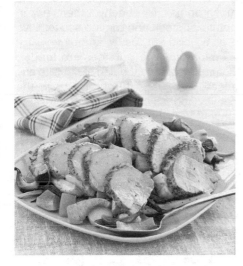

Ingredients

4 medium parsnips, quartered
lengthways
1 butternut squash (about 650g/1lb 7oz),
peeled, seeded and cut into chunks
2 red onions, each cut into 8 wedges
1 tbsp olive oil
grated zest of 1 lemon
2 tbsp pork seasoning or dried mixed
Italian herbs
500g/1lb 2oz lean pork tenderloin, in one
or two pieces
1 medium cooking apple
400ml/14fl oz chicken stock

1 Preheat the oven to 200C/gas 6/
fan 180C. Put the vegetables into a
roasting pan. Drizzle with the olive oil,
season with salt and pepper, then toss
everything together.

2 On a plate, mix together the lemon
zest and pork seasoning or herbs. Roll
the pork in the mixture then put it on top
of the vegetables. Roast for 40 minutes.
3 Peel and core the apple and cut it
into chunks. Scatter it into the roasting
tin, then pour in the stock and cook for a
further 15-20 minutes. Slice the pork,
arrange on a platter with the vegetables
then spoon over the pan juices.

Per serving

397 kcalories
Protein 34g
Carbohydrate 45g
Fat 10g
Saturated fat 2g
Fibre 12g
Added sugar none
Salt 0.85g

Fish pie with swede and potato topping

Making fish pie can be a bit of a palaver.
Not this one though, it's reassuringly
simple, using a tub of low-fat soft cheese
as the base for the sauce.
Takes 1 hour to 1 hour 15 minutes.
Serves 4.

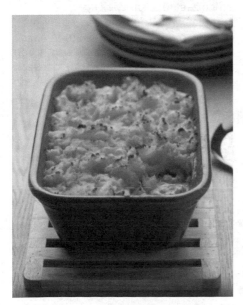

Ingredients

1 medium swede (weighing about
600g/1lb 5oz), cut into chunks
500g/1lb 2oz floury potatoes, cut into
chunks
200g tub low-fat soft cheese with garlic
and herbs
150ml/1/4 pint vegetable stock
4 tsp cornflour, blended with 2 tbsp cold
water
500g/1lb 2oz skinless, boneless cod, cut
into large chunks
140g/5oz smoked haddock, skinned and
cut into large chunks
85g/3oz cooked peeled prawns
1 tbsp chopped fresh parsley

1 Cook the swede and potatoes in
boiling, lightly salted water until tender –
about 20 minutes. Preheat the oven to
190C/gas 5/fan 170C.
2 Whilst the potatoes are cooking, put
the soft cheese and stock into a large
saucepan and heat gently, stirring with a
wooden spoon, until blended and
smooth. Now add the blended cornflour

and cook until thick. Gently stir the
chunks of fish into the sauce with the
prawns and parsley. Season with some
pepper, but don't add any salt, as the
smoked haddock and prawns add a
salty taste.
3 Tip the mixture into a 1.5 litre/
2 3/4 pint ovenproof baking dish. Drain the
swede and potatoes and mash them
well, seasoning with a few grindings of
black pepper. Spoon the mash on top of
the fish mixture to cover it completely.
Bake for 25-30 minutes until piping hot,
then transfer to a hot grill for a few
minutes to brown the top. Serve with
frozen, cooked peas or sweetcorn.

Per serving

354 kcalories
Protein 44g
Carbohydrate 36g
Fat 5g
Saturated fat none
Fibre 5g
Added sugar none
Salt 1.9g

Goulash in a dash

Takes 30 mins.
Serves 4.

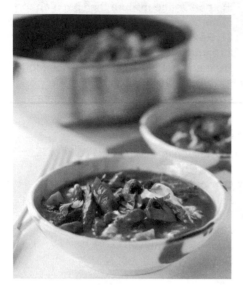

Ingredients

1 tbsp vegetable oil
300g/10oz stir-fry beef strips or minute steak cut into strips
100g/4oz chestnut mushrooms, quartered
2 tsp paprika
500g/1lb 2oz potatoes, peeled and cut into smallish chunks
600ml/1pt hot beef stock (a cube is fine)
500g jar tomato-based cooking sauce
Handful parsley leaves, roughly chopped
Natural bio yogurt, to serve

1 Heat half the oil in a large non-stick pan and fry the beef for 2 mins, stirring once halfway through. If your pan is small, do this in two batches. Tip the meat onto a plate. Heat the remaining oil in the pan (no need to clean) and fry the mushrooms for 2-3 mins until they start to colour.

2 Sprinkle the paprika over the mushrooms, fry briefly, then tip in potatoes, stock and tomato sauce. Give it all a good stir, cover and simmer for 20 mins until the potatoes are tender. Return the beef to the pan along with any juices, and warm through. Stir in the parsley and a swirl of yogurt, then serve straight from the pan.

Per serving

299 kcalories
Protein 23g
Carbohydrate 33g
Fat 9g
Saturated fat 2g
Fibre 3g
Added sugar 5g
Salt 1.59g

Healthy fish & chips with tartare sauce

Takes 40 to 45 minutes.
Serves 2.

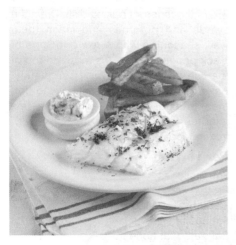

Ingredients

450g/1lb potatoes, peeled and cut into chips
1 tbsp olive oil, plus a little extra for brushing
2 white fish fillets, about 140g/5oz each
Grated zest and juice 1 lemon
Small handful parsley leaves, chopped
1 tbsp capers, chopped
2 heaped tbsp 0% Greek yogurt
Lemon wedge, to serve

1 Heat the oven to 200C/fan 180C/gas 6. Toss chips in oil. Spread over a baking sheet in an even layer, bake for 40 mins until browned and crisp. Put the fish in a shallow dish, brush lightly with oil, salt and pepper. Sprinkle with half the lemon juice, bake for 12-15 mins, after 10 mins sprinkle over a little parsley and lemon zest to finish cooking.

2 Meanwhile, mix the capers, yogurt, remaining parsley and lemon juice together, set aside and season if you wish. To serve, divide the chips between plates, lift the fish onto the plates and serve with a spoonful of yogurt mix.

Per serving

373 kcalories
Protein 35g
Carbohydrate 41g
Fat 9g
Saturated fat 1g
Fibre 3g
Added sugar none
Salt 0.96g

Vegetable balti

Takes 1 hour 20 to 1 hour 40 minutes.
Serves 4.

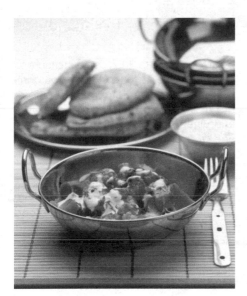

Ingredients

1 tbsp vegetable oil
1 large onion, thickly sliced
1 large garlic clove, crushed
1 apple, peeled, cored and cut into chunks
3 tbsp balti curry paste
1 medium butternut squash, peeled and cut into chunks
2 large carrots, thickly sliced
200g/8oz turnips, cut into chunks
1 medium cauliflower, weighing about 500g/1lb 2oz, broken into florets
400g can chopped tomatoes
425ml/3/4 pint hot vegetable stock
4 tbsp chopped fresh coriander, plus extra
150g pot low fat natural yogurt

1 Heat the oil in a large lidded pan, add the onion, garlic and apple and cook gently, stirring, for 5-8 minutes or until softened. Stir in the curry paste.

2 Tip in the fresh vegetables, add the tomatoes, stock and 3 tbsp of the coriander. Bring to the boil, cover, and then simmer for half an hour.

3 Remove lid and cook for 20 minutes until the liquid has reduced. Season.

4 Mix remaining coriander with the yogurt. Ladle the curry into bowls, top with the yogurt mixture and extra coriander. Serve with warm naan bread.

Per serving

201 kcalories
Protein 11g
Carbohydrate 25g
Fat 7g
Saturated fat 1g
Fibre 7g
Added sugar none
Salt 1.13g

Spaghetti with lemon, parmesan and peas

Takes 20 to 30 minutes.
Serves 2.

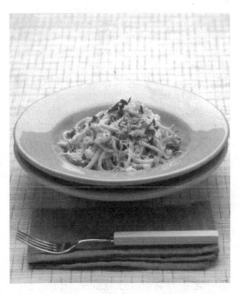

Ingredients

140g/5oz spaghetti
100g/4oz frozen petits pois or garden peas
2 tsp olive oil
1 small onion, finely chopped
100g/4oz low-fat soft cheese with chives and onion
Finely grated zest of 1 lemon
3 tbsp finely grated parmesan
1 tbsp chopped fresh flatleaf parsley

1 Bring a large pan of lightly salted water to the boil. Feed in the spaghetti and cook for about 10-12 minutes, until just tender. (Check the pack instructions for timings – 'quick cook' spaghetti takes only 3 minutes.) Add the peas for the last 2-3 minutes.

2 At the same time, heat the olive oil in a saucepan and fry the onion gently until softened and cooked, but not brown. Stir in the soft cheese and warm it through, adding 3 tbsp of the pasta cooking water to thin it down. Now stir in the lemon zest and 2 tbsp of the parmesan.

3 Drain the spaghetti and peas really well, return them to the pan and gently stir in the sauce. Season with salt and pepper, and then pile it into 2 serving bowls. Sprinkle the parsley and the remaining parmesan over the top and serve right away, with a mixed leaf salad.

Per serving

420 kcalories
Protein 22g
Carbohydrate 61g
Fat 11g
Saturated fat 3g
Fibre 5g
Added sugar none
Salt 0.83g

5 Alcohol and losing weight

1 With all the information about diet and exercise it is easy to forget about the role of alcohol in weight problems. All types of alcoholic drinks contain calories, and if you want to lose weight then it makes sense to think about your drinking.

2 The strength of different drinks can be compared using units of alcohol. A pint of beer (3.5% ABV) contains 2 units of alcohol, and a pint of stronger beer (5% ABV) nearly 3 units. A small glass of wine (12% ABV) contains about 1.5 units; and a bottle of wine 9-11 units, depending on strength.

3 Each unit of alcohol contains about 55 calories. However, because of its high carbohydrate content, beer contains significantly more calories than other drinks with about 91 calories per unit. A pint of beer (3.5% ABV) therefore contains 182 calories, or nearly one tenth of the total daily energy requirements for a man. Over a week, drinking 3 pints of beer a day adds up to a total of 3,350 calories, which equals the amount

Container	ABV	Units
Large glass of wine (175 mls)	15%	3
Small glass of wine (125 mls)	12%	1 1/2
Bottle of wine (750 mls)	12%	9
Pint of beer	5%	3
Pint of beer	3.5%	2
Single measure spirits (25 mls)	40%	1
Single measure spirits (35 mls)	40%	1 1/2

of calories needed to lose 1lb of weight. Therefore someone cutting their intake by 3 pints per day could expect to lose 1lb a week, without changing the amount that they eat or exercise. For you, this amount of beer may not be an issue, although cutting the amount of alcohol (particularly beer) that you drink will help you to reduce your calorie intake, and will always help you lose weight.

4 Alcohol is also important because it strongly affects hunger and appetite. It has a direct action on the stomach, stimulating it to relax and produce more gastric juices. Although there are a lot of calories present, particularly in beer, the stomach isn't able to tell this. Therefore it won't feel full in the way that it would after a meal, even if there is the same calorie content. Drinking, particularly on an empty stomach, makes blood sugar levels drop, which can sometimes cause almost uncontrollable feelings of hunger. Alcohol also affects areas of the brain that control behaviour, tending to cause a loss of inhibition and self-control. Put these factors together, and there is the risk of doing things when drunk that you'd never do when sober – as experienced by anyone who has ever eaten a dodgy late-night kebab after the pub.

5 However, in moderation, alcohol is safe and healthy, and can be an enjoyable part of a balanced lifestyle. Research has even shown that moderate drinkers have lower rates of illness than non-drinkers: the ideal intake for best health seems to be up to 10 units per week. The risk of health problems then steadily increases with increasing alcohol consumption. The recommended maximum intake for men is 3-4 units per day (for women 2-3 units per day). Major problems become much more likely with an intake of over 35 units per week for men (over 28 units for women).

6 It can be helpful to keep a drink diary. Keep a note of every alcoholic drink that you have, ideally over a two week period.

If you drink spirits, then use a measure to check the size of your drinks. If you drink wine, beer or cider, etc, make a note of the ABV%. Also make a note of where and when you have each drink – at the end of the fortnight you can check out the pattern of your drinking and work out your total intake in units.

7 In excess, alcohol can cause a wide range of physical problems such as poor erections, liver disease, high blood pressure, pancreatitis, diabetes, heart disease and cancer.

8 Drinking is also strongly linked to depression, anxiety and sleeping problems. Alcohol has a two-stage effect on the brain: the first effect is relaxation, loss of inhibition and a mild euphoria over a period of a few hours. However it then increases levels of stress, anxiety and depression the next day. Using alcohol to relieve these unpleasant feelings will steadily make them worse. Safety is also an issue, as more than half of all fatal car accidents, falls or drownings are alcohol-related. Nearly half of all injuries seen in casualty departments are linked to alcohol, either as a result of accident or violence.

9 Alcohol can also cause work problems, financial worries and damage relationships with partners, friends and families.

10 Alcohol may be a problem if you feel annoyed by people criticising your drinking, if you feel bad or guilty about your drinking, or if you have a drink first thing in the morning to steady your nerves (or get rid of a hangover). If you are worried about your drinking, sources of further help and advice would include:

• Your GP, who should be able to advise you further, check out your physical health, and can put you in touch with local sources of help.

• Drinkline (contact details below) offers information and self-help materials, help to callers worried about their own

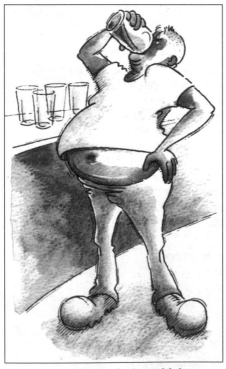

Beer is full of calories which go straight to your waist

drinking, support to the family and friends of people who are drinking, and advice to callers on where to go for help.
- Alcohol Concern (contact details below) has a useful website, with a services directory for information on how to access local alcohol services across the UK.
- Alcoholics Anonymous (contact details below).

Finally, some suggestions

- Walk, or cycle, to the pub – burn off some of the extra calories on the way.
- If you're thirsty, you'll tend to drink more – drink plenty of water, both during the day and when drinking alcohol. Alcohol tends to cause dehydration – try alternating glasses of alcoholic drink with glasses of water.
- Try to drink after a meal rather than before – you won't feel so hungry when you're eating, and you won't feel like drinking so much after your meal.
- Try cutting down the strength of what you drink: for example if you drink beer that is 5% ABV, try reducing it to 3.5% ABV.
- Try to have at least one alcohol-free day per week – if you can manage this comfortably, then you could try to have two or more alcohol-free days per week.
- Look for alternative activities to do with friends, partners or family that don't involve drinking – for example, meet up for a sports session, or go out to the movies instead.

Further information

11 If you would like to know more, look in the Contacts section at the back of the book, or contact:

For an on-line alcohol unit calculator
Website: www.projects.ex.ac.uk/trol/scol/ccalcoh2.htm

Drinkline
Offers information and self-help materials, help to callers worried about their own drinking, support to the family and friends of people who are drinking,

and advice to callers on where to go for help.
Tel: 0800 917 8282 (freephone)

Alcohol Concern
Has a useful website, with a services directory for information on how to access local alcohol services across the UK.
Website: www.alcoholconcern.org.uk

Alcoholics Anonymous
Tel: 0845 769 7555 (local rate calls)

6 Surgery – the last resort

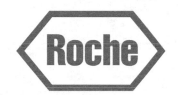

1 Sometimes it seems that nothing works, or if it does it's too little, or only a temporary fix. Sometimes a major overhaul is the only solution.

2 Weight loss surgery isn't for everyone; only around 500 operations are carried out in the UK each year, and only after other methods of losing weight, including diet, lifestyle advice, and usually drugs, have been exhausted. Individuals considering surgery have to undergo batteries of examinations, tests, medical and psychological screening before being deemed suitable to go under the knife. For these people the last voluntary act of weight control they will perform is signing the consent form, after which they hand over complete control of their weight to someone else for the first time ever; a team of surgeons, anaesthetists and nurses.

3 Surgery is indeed a drastic step to take, but sometimes desperate situations need desperate remedies, and so-called Bariatric surgery can be life

saving. It is normally available to people with a BMI of over 40, or 35 with severe illnesses related to obesity, and only those who have tried everything else first. Operations such as jaw wiring no longer exist, and liposuction doesn't count. These days surgery is so advanced that surgeons can use laparoscopic, or 'keyhole' techniques to avoid opening up the whole belly. There are two different types of operation:
- Restrictive, which restrict the size of the stomach using staples or bands, drastically reducing the amount of food it is possible to eat.
- Malabsorptive, in which a large part of the bowel is removed or by-passed, so although food can be eaten, it cannot be absorbed from the gut.

4 The two types of operation can also be combined.

5 Life after surgery is never the same again. It makes a big difference being unable to eat more than a couple of mouthfuls of soft, easily digestible food without suffering pain, bloating, vomiting and regurgitating. Mealtimes are completely different, and social evenings unrecognisable. But the advantage is that weight loss is dramatic, and permanent, as the operation is not reversed. Patients who have had surgery can expect to lose around 50% of their excess weight, and subsequent improvement in cholesterol, blood pressure, diabetes, etc.

6 Other procedures include placing an inflatable balloon in the stomach which gives the impression of fullness; and a gastric pacing device, which is implanted near the stomach, and stimulates the nerve supply, making the brain believe that a complete meal has been eaten.

7 Obese individuals undergoing any sort of surgery have increased risks under the anaesthetic, especially of lung problems and respiratory infections. It is advisable to be as fit as possible prior to undergoing an operation.

Chapter 3
Exercise

Contents

1 Myths and legends

MYTH: Sit ups will flatten your stomach

TRUTH: Abdominal exercises, such as sit-ups (crunches), are important for strengthening those muscles and improving posture. But muscle is muscle and fat is fat. If you have excess fat in your abdomen, you won't be able to see the muscles, no matter how many crunches you do. There's no such thing as spot reducing – losing weight in one specially designated area. To lose fat, you need to eat fewer calories than you burn.

MYTH: To do you any good, exercise has to be strenuous

TRUTH: You don't have to push yourself to extremes to get the health benefits of exercise. In fact, if you exercise excessively, you run the risk of overdoing it and ending up feeling worse. Alternate more strenuous workouts with easier ones (eg, a hilly walk one day that pushes you, followed by a flat, slower walk the next day).

MYTH: Going to a gym is the only way to get fit

TRUTH: People are more likely to stick with a home-based exercise programme. You can build in a considerable amount of activity into your daily life. Walking, dancing, cycling and gardening are all excellent activities that, if done regularly, will soon help you back to fitness. Plan a home workout doing things you enjoy. Lift some hand weights or cans of food while you watch your favourite TV show. It all counts.

MYTH: "No pain, no gain"

TRUTH: Exercise shouldn't hurt. A little muscle soreness when you do something new isn't unusual, but soreness doesn't equal pain. Learn to recognise the difference between discomfort and pain. You don't need to make your muscles burn to know they're working. If it hurts, stop doing it.

Many people new to exercise stop at the first feeling of breathing deeper or sweating because they think this is not normal. This is how the body naturally responds to exercise. But if you are gasping for breath or feel pain, stop and consult your doctor.

MYTH: Exercise makes you hungry

TRUTH: Exercise such as a brisk walk or run usually suppresses appetite, at least for a while. Swimming, because it lowers your core temperature, can leave you feeling hungry. Resist the urge to pile on the calories you have just burned and choose foods that release energy slowly such as unrefined carbohydrates rather than high sugar or fatty foods.

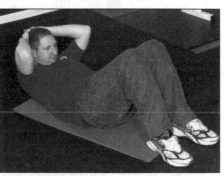

Sit-ups (crunches) are important for strengthening abdominal muscles and improving posture

2 Physical Activity

Get your motor running

1 The human body is an amazing piece of evolutionary engineering. Each joint and muscle is designed to work smoothly and effectively, governed by a complex control system (the central nervous system) and lubricated and fuelled by a cocktail of chemical reactions. On the whole, the body is quite remarkable in its ability to adapt to physical tasks and react to the demands we make of it. It is usually only through our own neglect that things start to go wrong. The human body evolved for movement. This century has seen us do everything we can to remove the need for movement from our lives. The combustion engine has taken away much of our need for walking from A to B. We invented moving staircases to make it easier for us to climb. Power tools, household appliances, lifts and the like all make for an easier life, but at the expense of our physical fitness. Two million years of evolutionary history, fine tuning the human body to run, chase, hunt, fish, carry and climb have been overturned in just one century. And the human body is struggling with this new role. It is simply not used to being so inactive. This, together with an abundance of high calorie, cheap food, is the reason why, as a nation, we're all getting so fat. It has been said that if we had to hunt, grow or gather everything that we eat, then, just as in the days of our cavemen ancestors, obesity would be unknown.

2 Many people blame our diet for the current rise in obesity, but that is only one side of the story. People put on weight when the amount of food they consume exceeds the amount of energy they expend. It really is as simple as that. Too many calories in and not enough out. You only have to look back at our grandparents to see that their very active lives kept them slim. The average post-war diet was just as high in calories as ours is today, but the lack of labour-saving devices meant that they burned off all these calories in their everyday lives. It was very common for people to grow their own food so many hours would be spent digging the garden. Car ownership was a fraction of what it is today so people would walk or cycle to work. For our grandmothers, simply having to hand-wash clothes or beat dust from carpets would work up a sweat and burn off excess calories.

6 out of 10 men in the UK are not active enough to benefit their health.

3 Many studies support the idea that it is not just our diet that is contributing to our weight gain, but also our low physical activity levels.

It creeps up on you!

The latest evidence suggests that being physically active throughout life can help maintain a healthy weight and prevent the 'creeping' weight gain that occurs as we get older. The body tends to slow down a little with age, which means that we expend fewer calories as we get older. It doesn't take much to gain weight, just eating 50 kcals (equivalent to a digestive biscuit) a day more than we expend will lead to a weight gain of approximately 2 kg a year. At this rate, within 10 years, a healthy weight person can quite easily become obese. On the other hand, just expending 50 kcals a day more than we consume will lead to weight loss or, at the very least, ensure that a healthy weight is maintained.

Healthy weight:
energy in = energy out

Get it off – keep it off!

Studies have shown that the combination of a reduced calorie diet and increased physical activity is much more effective in achieving weight loss than diet alone. Furthermore, people who exercise as part of their weight loss programme are much less likely to regain lost weight.

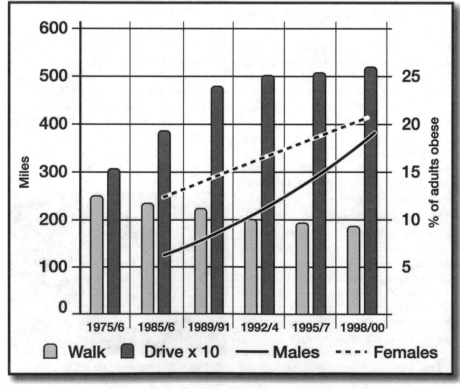

Distance travelled by walking or car and obesity

Combine a healthy diet with physical activity for best results

Using physical activity alone (that is without dieting) to reduce obesity, exercise programmes would need to prescribe an energy expenditure of 3000-3500 kcals per week. That is equivalent to approximately 45-60 minutes of purposeful walking performed at a moderate intensity (70% of maximum heart rate) on most days of the week.
Ross and Jansen 2001

4 If you're trying to lose weight, then physical activity is your greatest ally. The chances are that you know that you need to get exercising to shift those extra pounds, but what does that really mean? The thought of getting togged up in exercise gear is enough to put most people off before they even start. But being more active doesn't necessarily mean signing up to the local aerobics class or joining the gym. There are many other ways of building physical activity into your life.

Definitions

Exercise

This usually refers to a structured session of physical activity taken at a specific time and performed to enhance health and well-being.

Physical activity

This could be any activity, at work, during leisure time or in the home, which uses large muscle groups (such as the leg muscles) and contributes to energy expenditure. It can include structured exercise sessions.

5 Just because you are not taking part in structured exercise sessions, like playing football or going to the gym, this does not mean that you cannot be physically active. Experts say that, in order to maintain health, we should all aim to be physically active for at least 30 minutes on most days of the week. Many people would argue that to be truly 'fit', we should be doing at least three vigorous exercise sessions a week ON TOP of the 30 minutes of physical activity a day. But let's not run before we can walk. If you have been inactive for a long time, or if you are overweight, you need to build up your activity level gradually and be realistic about how much you can do and fit into your lifestyle.

Are you getting enough?

Current guidelines from the Department of Health state that 'adults should have 30 minutes of moderate activity (such as walking, cycling, gardening) on at least 5 days of the week'.

Why bother?

6 If you are cutting down on your calorie intake, then the chances are, you are probably starting to lose weight already. So why bother to be more physically active? The fact is that active people live longer, have fewer health problems, are less likely to be overweight, have more energy and are usually happier than inactive people.

7 The reason that the Government is so keen for us all to be more active is because there is now a huge amount of evidence to suggest that physical activity can improve health in many different ways. The National Heart Forum says that if everyone walked a minimum of 30 minutes, five days a week, 37 per cent of heart attacks could be prevented and millions of pounds could be saved each year.

8 But it's not just your heart that benefits from exercise, there are many other effects. As well as reducing the

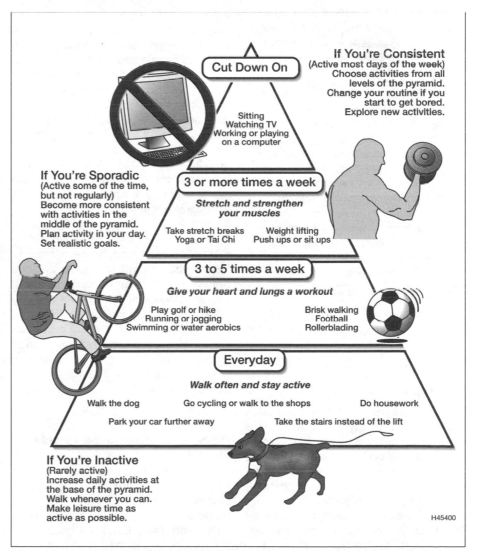

The Activity Pyramid: each week, try to balance your physical activity using this guide

chances of having a heart attack, regular physical activity can help prevent stroke, diabetes, some cancers – particularly bowel cancer – lower blood pressure and improve your cholesterol level. It can help prevent osteoporosis (brittle bone disease), boost the immune system (making it less likely for you to catch common viruses like colds and flu), give you more energy and even improve your sex life. In addition to this it will make your muscles stronger and more flexible and make you less likely to suffer from depression. Phew! The person who invents a pill that can do all this will be richer than Bill Gates!

Regular exercise can improve your sex life, but sex in itself can count as physical activity. The missionary position (you on top) burns around 8 kcals a minute – the same as a brisk walk.

Study results show that even in people who are overweight, their risk of heart disease is reduced if they achieve a moderate level of fitness compared with people who are overweight and unfit. In addition, regardless of whether you lose weight or not, regular physical activity is associated with improvements in blood pressure, lower blood sugar levels and lower cholesterol levels.

3 How does exercise work?

Heart health

1 Physical activity helps improve heart health in many ways. The heart is a muscle, just like the biceps or any other muscle in your body. The more it is used, the stronger it gets. Exercise makes the heart beat faster but also, over time, makes it beat more efficiently. In other words, the heart pumps out more blood with every heart beat. A more efficient heart means that it can perform the same work at a lower heart rate. This is what is called a 'training effect' and can lead to a

lower resting pulse. Exercise also reduces the stickiness of the blood which helps reduce clots and improve circulation. Being overweight increases the workload on the heart, but not in the beneficial way that exercise does.

Diabetes

2 Diabetes occurs when there is an imbalance between blood sugar (glucose) and insulin in the body. Glucose is the simple form of carbohydrates that give us energy, insulin is a hormone that helps control blood sugar levels and is produced in special cells in the pancreas. When glucose levels rise, extra insulin is produced to remove this glucose and store it in the liver. When there is insufficient insulin being produced, diabetes can occur. Diabetes is more common in people who are overweight or obese. Type I diabetes tends to occur in young people and the exact cause of this is unknown, but may be associated with a virus that destroys insulin-producing cells. Type II diabetes is more common and tends to occur in people over 40 and its onset may be gradual. Excess body fat can decrease the body's sensitivity to insulin. Diabetes can be diagnosed during a routine medical examination by having your doctor look at sugar levels in your urine.

3 Physical activity can help by helping to reduce the amount of body fat and by increasing the body's sensitivity to insulin, thereby redressing the balance between glucose and insulin levels. If you are diabetic, it is important that you take certain precautions when you exercise in order to prevent a sudden drop in glucose levels, which can lead to dizziness or fainting and confusion. Diabetes can also lead to poor circulation, so it is important to check your feet for any signs of cuts or infection.

Physical activity helps reduce cholesterol

4 Physical activity has been shown to increase the amount of 'good' cholesterol in the blood. Cholesterol is made up of Low Density Lipoproteins (LDL) and High Density Lipoproteins (HDL). LDL is the 'bad' sort that clogs your arteries and leads to clots and high blood pressure. HDL is the 'good'

cholesterol which actually has a 'scouring' effect on the arteries. Exercise increases the amount of HDL in the blood.

Helps prevent cancer

5 No one would disagree that smoking causes cancer, but it is now thought that being inactive can also substantially increase your risk of developing the disease. It is estimated that 1 in 10 cancers are obesity related. Obesity is associated with being inactive. It is still unclear as to how exercise actually helps prevent cancer, but studies are beginning to show a consistent link between activity and reduced risk of cancer. In particular, one study showed that the risk of developing cancer of the bowel can be halved with regular exercise. The mechanism for this is still unclear, but it may be simply that more active people have a more efficient digestive system which means that food travels through the body quicker. Higher insulin levels have been shown to trigger the growth of some cancer cells. Regular exercise, by decreasing the amount of body fat, can help reduce insulin levels, therefore reducing you risk of cancer.

How physical activity affects the immune system

6 Moderate levels of regular exercise have been shown to enhance the immune system, helping it to fight off illness and reduce the incidence of infection. Exercise can also be used to aid recovery from illness or surgery. Being active increases your blood flow and raises the oxygen levels, helping to repair damaged tissue. Exercise has also been shown to increase the number of 'natural killer' (or NK) cells in the body. These NK cells constantly monitor the areas germs can enter, such as the nose and lungs and digestive tract. NK cells immediately destroy any cells they do not recognise, thereby protecting us against a large number of infectious organisms.

Strengthens bones, makes you stronger and more flexible

7 Studies have shown that people who are active when they are young amass a reserve of bone mineral that may help to prevent the onset of osteoporosis in older age. But exercising at any age has been shown to slow down the loss of

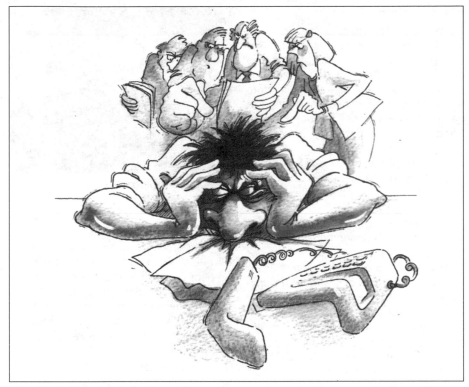

Exercise also helps to reduce stress and can help us cope better with everyday problems

bone mass that starts to occur in your 30s and 40s. In some cases is not only halts the decline, but can actually reverse it. You are much less likely to suffer from brittle bone disease if you take regular exercise.

8 The first astronauts to spend time in space experienced significant loss of bone density. This is because in space you are weightless and there is no load on your muscles and bones. Strong muscles and strong bones go hand in hand. If your muscles are strong you can lift heavier weights. Lifting heavy weights puts stress on the bones and it is this stress that stimulates the bone and makes it stronger. Now astronauts prevent this loss of bone density by exercising for several hours a day as part of their preparation programme before going into space.

9 By the age of 65, people who don't exercise will lose between 30 and 40 percent of their muscle power. But strength can be improved at any age and studies have shown that weight training programmes, even in your 80s, can at least double muscle power.

10 Stronger muscles mean you are less prone to injury, but only if the muscle is flexible too. Exercising and being active means that your muscles are regularly taken through their full range of movement, which keeps them flexible. Your joints, just like any moving part in a machine, will benefit from regular activity. When you are active your joints are lubricated by fluid (this fluid is called synovial fluid and is found in most joints) which ensures they move smoothly and easily. When you are inactive, your body's joints will start to seize up, just as a mechanical joint that is not kept oiled will rust.

Exercise and mental health

11 As well as being good for the body, physical activity is also good for the mind. Active people are less likely to suffer from depression and anxiety. Doctors actually recommend exercise as a treatment for mild and moderate depression and it can, for some people, be as effective as anti-depressant drugs. If you are feeling anxious, getting out for a brisk walk or exercising can alleviate much of those feelings. Exercise also helps to reduce stress and can help us cope better with everyday problems.

4 So you want to get fit?

1 The chances are, if you are reading this, you have at least given some thought to becoming more active. Before you embark on this journey to better health, you need to prepare yourself. If you've been inactive for many years, then it is important to get an idea of your current level of fitness and health before you start. Think of it as putting your vehicle through a service. This will help identify any potential problems that might impede your journey and enable you to take action to put them right. It is a good idea to check with your doctor before you increase the amount of physical activity that you do or before starting an exercise programme. Take a look at the questions below. If you have answered 'yes' to one or more of them, then discuss your plans with your doctor before you start.

2 This questionnaire is designed to help you decide whether you are physically ready to take up more exercise. Answering 'yes' to any of these questions does not necessarily mean that you cannot become more active, but you may need to check with your doctor so that he can help you structure a safe and effective programme.

- *Has your doctor ever said that you have a heart condition or have you every experienced a stroke or blood clot?*
- *Do you every experience pain in your chest when you are physically active or at any other time?*
- *Do you ever feel faint, lose your balance or lose consciousness?*
- *Do you have a bone or joint condition such as rheumatoid arthritis?*
- *Is your doctor currently prescribing medication for high blood pressure or a heart condition?*
- *Have you had surgery in the last three months?*
- *Do you suffer from epilepsy that is hard to control?*
- *Do you suffer from diabetes?*

3 It is very unlikely that your doctor will tell you that you cannot increase your activity level. Very few conditions are made worse with exercise. In fact most physical conditions are improved with regular physical activity. The important thing is to select the right exercise for you and build up gradually. You might not be able to go straight back to playing a full 90 minutes for your local footie team, but it is unlikely that you won't be able to increase the amount of walking you do or start an exercise programme at your local gym.

Fitness Tests

4 Don't skip the questionnaire above, it will give you valuable information about your readiness to exercise. If you have answered 'yes' to any of the questions, check with your GP (doctor) before starting your new programme. If it has been a long time since you took any meaningful exercise, it is always a good idea to get a check up before you start.

5 If you join a gym, then the staff there will probably ask you to complete a very similar questionnaire. A good gym will also recommend that you check with your doctor before starting a new exercise programme if you answer 'yes' to any of the questions. Be suspicious of any gym that does not ask you about your health history.

6 If there are no reasons why you should not be more active or your doctor has told you that you are fine to start exercising more, then you may want to consider testing your current level of fitness before you start. Knowing your fitness level will help you in selecting the right exercise for you and also give you a benchmark for monitoring your progress as you become fitter. It can also help you set realistic goals. Knowing where you are starting from makes it a lot easier to plan your journey to better health.

Before you start your new physical activity or exercise programme, it is a good idea to consult your doctor to make sure your are ready to increase the amount of exercise you take. Fitness tests can be useful for monitoring your progress, although some people can find them de-motivating. Speak to an exercise professional who will be able to help you ascertain your readiness to exercise, both from a physical and psychological perspective.

What is fitness?

7 Health professionals agree that there are three main dimensions to physical fitness. The first of these is cardiovascular fitness and is sometimes called aerobic fitness or stamina. It refers to the ability of your heart and lungs to deal with physical activity or exercise. Secondly, experts recognise musculoskeletal strength as an essential component of fitness. This refers to the strength within your bones and joints and yours muscles. Thirdly, flexibility is considered to be an important dimension to fitness. Many experts now agree that there is a fourth dimension to physical fitness, that of metabolic fitness, or your body's ability to deal with metabolising (or processing) fats and sugars. People who are unfit are more likely to suffer with high cholesterol and diabetes. All these components can be improved with increased physical activity or exercise. These improvements are known as a 'training effect' and can be measured using a variety of tests.

Tests you can do yourself at home

8 Although you may want to consider having some aspects of your fitness monitored by a professional, there are many ways you can assess your current level of fitness and monitor your progress at home. Being able to monitor your progress can really help to keep you motivated, but not everyone will want to be the subject of professional scrutiny. If you are too shy to join a gym then DIY tests are for you. Also, if you are the type of person who is quite self-motivated and keen to do a home-based programme, these tests will keep you on track.

Testing your heart rate

9 Cardiovascular fitness is the key to prolonging the length and quality of your life. As you become fitter, your hard becomes more efficient and is able to pump out more blood each time it beats. This means that the rate at which your heart beats will decrease with training. There is a marked difference between the resting heart rate (or pulse) of a trained athlete and an unfit person. The resting heart rate of an average adult is around 72 beats per minute. For an unfit person, this can be as high as 80 to 90

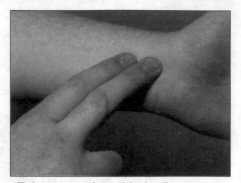

Take your pulse with the fingers not the thumb

beats per minute, whereas the heart of a very fit person may only need to beat at 50 beats per minute to deliver the same amount of blood to the rest of the body. Taking your resting heart rate will give you an indication of your fitness level and also enable you to chart your progress as you get fitter and your resting pulse decreases.

To take your resting pulse

10 Make sure you have been seated for at least 10 minutes. Avoid consuming caffeine before your test and ensure you are relaxed and calm. You may find it best to take your pulse first thing in the morning, before you get out of bed. When you come to repeat your test after three months, try to ensure that you take your pulse at the same time and under similar conditions as before. Find a watch with a second hand or a seconds counter. Place your index and middle fingers (not your thumb as this also has a pulse) on the inside of your wrist near the base of your thumb. Press gently and you should feel your pulse. Count the number of beats during 15 seconds and multiply this number by four. This will give you your resting heart rate in beats per minute (bpm). Note down your result and test yourself once you have been exercising regularly for at least 12 weeks. You should notice that your pulse is lower. You are on the right road to improving your health!

11 Another method for testing your heart rate involves using a heart rate monitor.

Rating of Perceived Exertion – how does it feel for you?

12 Instead of taking your heart rate during exercise, experts often use a system called the 'Rating of Perceived Exertion'. This system can be used at home to help you understand how hard you are working, but also to monitor how your fitness progresses as you exercise more. Knowing how 'it feels' when you are doing a particular exercise will help you understand how you respond to effort and encourages you to listen to your body. Using this system, you rate your effort level by how hard you think you are working. If you note your RPE at a given point in your exercise session, you should see that, over time, your perceived effort will be less than when you started your training programme. One way of using this scale is to find a set walk route, make a note of how long it takes you to complete it, and note your RPE at a given point in the walk. Of course, if you complete the walk in a quicker time, your RPE may be higher.

Using time, RPE and resting pulse, you can get a rough idea of improvements in your fitness. In addition to this, you should find that, over time and with regular physical activity, everyday activities become easier to perform. You'll probably notice that climbing stairs, playing with the kids or even your daily work leaves you less breathless and with more energy.

Rating of Perceived Exertion Scale

Numerical rating	Rating in Words	Sample Description
0	Nothing at all	Sitting still, reading
1	Very light	You are barely moving, maybe just standing at the bar
2	Light	Walking around the house, or strolling
3		
4		
5	Moderate	Walking at a moderate pace, gardening
6		
7	Hard	Cycling over rolling hills
8	Very hard	Walking at a fast pace
9		
10	Extremely hard	Walking at a brisk pace up a hill

5 Weighing-in

1 Let's not get too heavy about weight. For many of us, the prospect of stepping onto that pair of scales in the corner of the bathroom is something we dread. Although it can be useful to know how heavy you are, what you are actually measuring is the total weight of your organs, bones, blood, fat and muscle. What really matters is the amount of fat you are carrying, or your body composition. There are some scales on the market that do give you a measure of your fat percentage, by sending a small electrical current through your body and measuring the resistance in the body tissues. Fatty tissue blocks or impedes the electrical current or signal more than other body tissues. This is because fat has a very low water content, whereas muscle and other tissues contain 70 percent water (which is better at conducting electricity). These body fat scales are more informative than scales that only measure weight.

2 If you do weigh yourself, then remember that weight can fluctuate by as much as 5lb each day and that it will vary at different times of the day. Try to weigh yourself every two weeks, at the same time of day and with the same amount of clothing. Keep a record of your weight, but remember that muscle is heavier than fat, and if you are exercising more and building muscle, you may find that your weight does not drop as quickly as you had hoped. What you should notice however is a change in your shape. It is useful to keep a pair of 'reference' trousers, one pair you used to fit into and the ones you are currently wearing. Try them on each month to see how you are doing.

Waist to Hip ratio

3 Studies have found that men who have a waist-to-hip ratio greater than 1 have a higher risk of developing heart disease. Knowing your waist-to-hip ratio can be useful when trying to lose weight and is a simple test that can be done at home. All you need is a tape measure.

Measure your waist at the narrowest point then measure your hips at the widest point. Divide your waist measurement by your hip measurement. For example, if your waist measurement is 102 cm, and your hip measurement is 106 cm, you divide 102 by 106 which gives 0.96. Aim for a waist-to-hip ratio below 1 for good health.

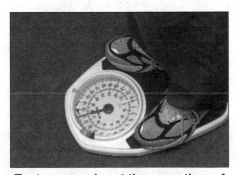
Try to use scales at the same time of the day, but not too often

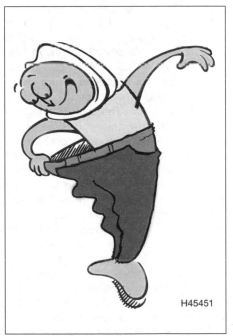
H45451
Keep a pair of 'reference' trousers to see how you are doing

Body Mass Index

4 If you have visited your doctor about your weight, he or she may have calculated your Body Mass Index (BMI) to ascertain whether you are overweight. Rather than just taking your overall weight, this calculation takes into account your height as well. It is a figure that is frequently used by insurance companies when estimating your health risk, but it does have its limitations. It does not tell you how much of your body is fat. Because muscle is heavier than fat, muscle-bound athletes can be labelled as 'overweight' because they carry more muscle than average for their heights (see Chapter 5 to calculate your BMI. If maths isn't your thing, there are plenty of websites which will calculate your BMI for you. Just search the web for 'calculating your BMI'. Alternatively, your doctor will help you calculate your BMI and help you to interpret the result). A BMI greater than 40 indicates a very strong risk of heart disease and other obesity related complications

Blood pressure

5 Before you step up the amount of exercise you do, it is a good idea to have your blood pressure checked by your doctor or a fitness professional. Home blood pressure measures can be inaccurate and a professional will be better placed to explain your tests results to you. Blood pressure gives an indication of how open your blood vessels are. It is usually given in two numbers as in 120 over 80 or 120/80. The first number relates to your systolic pressure and the second to your diastolic pressure. The systolic measure is the pressure within your vessels as your heart ejects blood and diastolic pressure is the pressure when your heart relaxes and prepares for its next pump. Ideally, blood pressure should be 120/80 or below. If it is higher than this, this indicates that your heart needs to work harder to pump the blood through your blood vessels. If your blood pressure is higher than 145/95 then you are suffering from hypertension. Discuss this with your GP who will be able to advise you. He may prescribe medication to help lower your blood pressure. Stress and caffeine can affect your reading, as well as apprehension about the test itself. This is sometimes referred to as 'white

coat syndrome'. Your doctor may recommend that you have your blood pressure taken again at a different time in order to get a more accurate reading. If you have high blood pressure, it is important that you build up the amount of exercise you do very gradually and do not over-exert yourself. Don't use this as an excuse not to exercise though, increasing the amount of physical activity you do, even if it is just walking more, will be beneficial and help to lower your blood pressure if done regularly.

Blood Pressure Categories for Adults*

Category	Systolic (mmHg)	Diastolic (mmHg)
Normal	<130	<85
High Normal	130-139	85-89
High Blood Pressure		
Stage 1	140-159	90-99
Stage 2	160-179	100-109
Stage 3	180-209	110-119
Stage 4	>= 210	>= 120

* For those not taking medicine for high blood pressure and not having a short-term serious illness.
< less than
>= greater than or equal to

Tests you can take in a gym or with a fitness professional

6 A good gym will offer you a comprehensive fitness assessment before you are shown how to use its facilities. One of the main advantages of joining a gym is that you will be safely guided through the process of getting fitter, from testing your current level of fitness, to devising an appropriate programme and adapting that programme as you get fitter. Before undertaking any fitness tests, you should be asked about your health history and complete a questionnaire similar to that in Section 4. If you answer 'yes' to any of the questions, or if it has been a long time since you took any meaningful exercise, you will be advised to seek your doctor's advice before you take the tests or increase the amount of exercise you do. It is in your interest to be honest with the gym staff about your health history to ensure that you are safe when exercising. It is unlikely that they will not be able to tailor a programme for your needs, but they cannot be responsible

for your failing to disclose a health problem.

7 A good fitness assessment will look at the three main components of fitness, that is cardiovascular fitness (how fit is your heart?), strength and flexibility. It will also involve an evaluation of your body composition, either by measuring your fat percentage or measuring your waist-to-hip ratio. If you are trying to lose weight, the fitness professional will also look at your diet and make recommendations about healthy eating. Be wary of any fitness professional that offers miracle solutions to lose weight. Remember that the only way to lose weight is to exercise more and take in fewer calories. Pills and potions that seem too good to be true are usually just that.

How fit is your heart?

8 Most reputable gyms or clubs will perform something called a sub-maximal test to estimate your aerobic capacity or cardiovascular fitness. These tests involve measuring your heart rate as you exercise on either a stationary bicycle or a treadmill at a level which is about 75 to 85 percent of your maximum effort (hence the name *sub*-maximal). Maximal tests – where you perform at your maximum effort to the point of near-exhaustion – should only be performed by a trained and qualified medical expert.

9 The fitness professional taking you through the test will advise you as to the most suitable apparatus for the test. If you are a cyclist, he may recommend the stationary bicycle, if you are a walker or runner, then the treadmill may be more suitable. Some clubs or academic institutions may be able to offer sub-maximal tests for disabled people, using hand cranks or apparatus that involves only the upper body.

10 You will be fitted with a heart rate monitor which is strapped around your chest and sends a signal to a watch or device on the cycle or treadmill displaying your heart rate. The test usually lasts around 15 minutes, during which time the tester will gradually increase the intensity by increasing the resistance on the cycle, or increasing the incline on the treadmill. The test should not be very hard and, for most people, unless they are very fit, is unlikely to

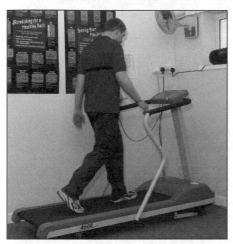

A heart rate monitor is strapped around your chest and sends a signal to a device on the cycle or treadmill displaying your heart rate

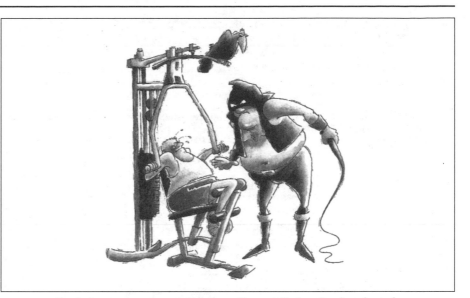

Tests to measure muscle strength usually involve hard work

involve running. A brisk walking pace on a slight incline on the treadmill should be sufficient to take the heart rate up to around 75 percent of its maximum. If you are very unfit, then your heart rate will reach this level even with a moderate paced walk. The fitness professional should give you a record of your results and schedule a second fitness evaluation in six weeks. The results of your test can be used to devise a tailor-made exercise programme.

11 Another commonly used test is a one-mile walk test. Again, using a heart rate monitor, you will be asked to walk a one mile course (or less if that is too much for you) as briskly as you can and your trainer will time your walk and make a note of your heart rate. The advantage of this test is that you can repeat it by yourself at any time using a heart rate monitor, once you have identified a suitable course.

Strength test

12 If you are joining a gym, it is likely that your trainer will include some strength training in your programme. With appropriate training, you can increase the strength and endurance of your muscles and increase their bulk. As we have said before, muscle is not just heavier than fat, but it also uses more energy than fat. By increasing the amount of lean muscle mass in your body, you increase your metabolic rate, which means that your body burns more

calories, even at rest. The two components to overall strength are muscular endurance and muscular strength. Muscular endurance refers to your muscles' ability to keep working over time, whereas muscular strength refers to the amount of force your muscles can exert in one try. Tests to measure strength usually consist of muscular endurance tests, where you will be asked to perform push-ups or a modified sit-up called a 'crunch'. Muscular strength is sometimes measured using a grip test where you squeeze a hand-held device as hard as you can.

13 These strength tests are not recommended for people who are very unfit or who have joint or back problems that could be made worse by the test. Your trainer will advise you as to suitable tests for you.

Flexibility

14 You may, depending on your level of fitness, be invited to perform a flexibility test, which involves sitting on the floor with your legs straight out in front of you and reaching forward with both arms towards your toes. The trainer will measure how far you can reach which will give you an indication of your flexibility in your hamstrings and your lower back. With regular stretching exercises and increased exercise, you should find that your flexibility improves and you become more supple.

Body composition tests

15 Because knowing your overall weight is of limited value, most gyms will offer a body composition test to ascertain how much of you is made up of fat. This can be done using a body fat monitoring device called a bioelectrical impedance monitor. Usually a small electrode is attached to your toe and another to your hand an electric signal is sent around your body. The more fat you have, the slower the signal because fat impedes the current.

16 Sometimes doctors and trainers use skinfold calipers to pinch your skin and fat away from the bone and muscle. Measurements are taken at several sites on the body, typically the back of the arm, below the shoulder on the back and just above the hip on the abdomen. These measurements are then fed into a

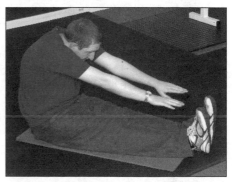

Measure how far you can reach to give an indication of the flexibility in your hamstrings and your lower back

formula that gives you your overall fat percentage. The accuracy of this type of test depends largely on the skill of the tester and in very overweight people may not be appropriate.

6 Selecting the right model – choosing the right physical activity for you

The basics

1 If you're a big bloke, there is no point in trying to squeeze yourself into a small performance car. Apart from being extremely uncomfortable, the chances are the seatbelt won't fit (or you won't fit behind the steering wheel) and you'll be unsafe as well. Choosing the right physical activity or exercise programme is just the same. If you aim for something too high powered, you'll find yourself struggling to keep up. Not only that, but you'll be running the risk of doing yourself serious damage. The best approach is to start with gentle, easy exercise that you enjoy and gradually build up. The biggest mistake that people make when they take up exercise is to aim too high. Be realistic about what you can achieve and don't underestimate the importance of simple exercise such as walking or cycling. Studies have shown that overweight people who use walking as their physical activity experienced greater weight loss and were more likely to stick with it.

Sticking with it

2 In choosing what type of exercise to take up, one of the most important things to consider is whether you think you can stick with it. The benefits of physical activity cannot be banked. Studies have shown that people who were athletes in their youth, but who subsequently gave up exercising, were just as much at risk of heart disease and related complications as those who never took regular exercise. On the other hand, people who took up exercise in later years and continued exercising regularly, had a better chance of surviving longer than the ex-athletes.

3 So remember:
- *You can't bank the benefits of physical activity.*
- *You need to do it regularly if it is to do you any good.*

Exercise is for life, not just for Christmas
One post-lunch walk on Christmas day will not stave off the heart attack.

Choose something you enjoy

4 With this in mind, it is important that you choose activities that you enjoy and that fit into your lifestyle. Just increasing the amount of activity in your everyday life can make a big difference. Ideally, aim for variety and as well as everyday activities, include some more structured sessions of play, walking, gym workouts or sport.

Build up gradually

5 Don't try to run before you can walk. If it has been a long time since you took any exercise, taking up jogging is likely to leave you exhausted and in pain. If the activity is too difficult or uncomfortable, you are much less likely to stick with it.

Fitting it in

6 Be realistic about how much time you can allocate to your activity. If you work long hours or do shift work, don't commit to a gym that has restricted opening hours. Try instead to build activity into your everyday life. Start by walking more by getting off the bus a stop earlier, or parking the car further away from the shops or workplace. Use the stairs rather than the lift or escalator. Do more housework and find the motivation to complete all those DIY jobs you've been putting off. As well as getting more exercise, you'll reap the benefit of a happy family!

It's the little things that make the big difference

If you overeat by just 100 kcals every day – the equivalent of a chocolate biscuit – then over 10 years, you will gain more than 45 kgs. Similarly, if you burn off just 100 kcals a day more than you consume – equivalent to just 20 minutes of cleaning the car, you will stave off the creeping obesity that occurs as our bodies slow down with age and maintain a healthy weight.

1kg fat = 7700 kcals

Calories burned with various activities

Activity	kcal burned in 20 minutes by a 90 kg man
Billiards	74
Bowling	172
Car washing	122
Mowing (not ride on!)	200
Plastering	138
Sawing by hand	218
Stacking firewood	156
Vacuuming	116
Walking – brisk 4 mph pace	174
Walking – moderate 3 mph pace	134
Welding	90
Window cleaning	106

How much? How often? How hard?

7 The current Government guidelines state that we should all be taking at least 30 minutes of physical activity on most days of the week. Although this may sound like a lot, it can be broken down into two 15 minutes sessions, or three 10 minute sessions. Any activity that leaves you feeling slightly warmer and breathing more deeply counts. Walking at a brisk pace is ideal for most people, but if you are very overweight or currently very inactive, you may find that even this is too much. Listen to your body and look for the stop signs (see box opposite).

Only 30% of people in the UK are currently active at the recommended level of 30 minutes on most days. This means that 70% do not take enough exercise to benefit their health.

---

8 If you really want to make a difference to your health and lose weight you will need to invest a little more time and energy. Experts agree that, in order to lose weight, people should aim to be active for 60 minutes at least three times a week, in addition to the 30 minutes of daily activity. So, as well as accruing your 30 minutes of daily activity, you should aim to include some more structured exercise sessions into your weekly total.

STOP SIGNS

It is quite natural to feel hot and sweaty during exercise and to be breathing much more heavily. This is usually a sign that you are working at the correct intensity. However, experiencing any of the following should act as a warning that you may be overdoing things.

Pain or discomfort

Expect to feel a little discomfort at first, especially if you are unused to physical activity, but any pain in the chest or upper body, particularly the left arm, is a sign to stop exercising and seek your doctor's advice.

Breathlessness

If you are finding it hard to control your breathing or gasping for breath and this does not subside as you decrease the intensity of your physical activity, stop and consult your doctor.

Fainting

If you faint during or just after exercise, seek your doctor's advice before continuing. If you experience dizziness or nausea during exercise, slow down and wait to see if it subsides. If it does not, then stop the activity.

Palpitations

A fast or irregular heartbeat is a danger signal.

---

9 If you are not yet active at the recommended level, don't panic, everyone has to start somewhere. Trying to do too much too soon will lead to you feeling burned out and exhausted and unlikely to stick with it. It is better to aim for a slower, steady pace and keep going for longer than pushing yourself too hard to start. Think 'tortoise' rather than 'hare'. Devise a plan of attack and stick with it. Once you are achieving the minimum amount of 30 minutes on most days, you can start to think about including other more structured activities and sports.

10 Thirty minutes of brisk walking every day will give you far more benefit than a weekly 20 minute game of squash or 10 minutes flat out on the football pitch on a Sunday morning. Taking exercise in this way is a bit like taking all your tablets at once.

Effortless exercise

11 Tips for increasing the amount of physical activity in your everyday life.

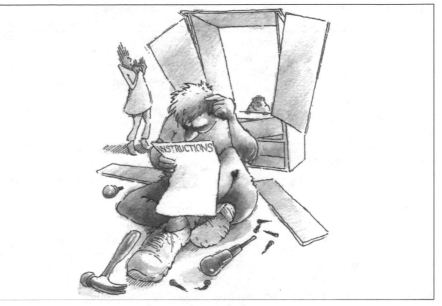

Put up those shelves

- Shift up a gear. Do everyday tasks at work and around the home with more gusto.
- Switch to manual. Whenever possible, chose the non-powered tool. Climb stairs rather than take the lift or escalator. Deliver messages in person rather than by e-mail. Park your car further away from the shops or your workplace and walk.
- Collect brownie points. Offer to do household chores, clean windows, vacuum. Put up those shelves, paint the hallway, give the car a service. All good calorie-burning DIY tasks...
- Go for a spin. Look for opportunities to have calorie-burning fun. Play with the kids. Chase a frisbee, kick a ball, surprise the dog with a long walk. Have more sex.
- Park up. On long journeys, park up at a local beauty spot and take a walk rather than snoozing in the cab. It will energise you and, if you need to sleep, help you sleep better.

7   Shifting up a gear – beyond the basics

Working out – it's time to get serious about exercise

1 Increasing the amount of physical activity in your daily life is the first step towards improving your health. If you really want to see results and win your fight with the flab, then you need to start building in regular structured exercise sessions. The same rules apply to structured exercise as to other forms of daily physical activity, in that you need to find something you enjoy, you need to build up the intensity gradually and you need to be able to do it regularly.

Experts recommend a minimum of 30 minutes of physical activity on most days. However, in order to lose weight, the recommendation is that you build in 60 minutes or more of physical activity on 3 days of the week.

Incidental Physical Activity – IPA

Your best mate in your fight to lose your gut! Don't neglect your best mate when you take up more structured exercise. It's great that you've chosen to take up a sport, go cycling, swimming, walking or going to the gym, but Incidental Physical Activity (IPA) is still your best friend when it comes to making a difference to your total calorie expenditure. Structured exercise sessions alone are unlikely to add up to 60 minutes 5 times a week, but adding more physical activity into your everyday life will ensure that you're really getting enough.

Exercise Basics

2 Although any activity is better than none, to really make a difference to your health and your fitness, you need to exercise at a level which is going to challenge your heart and lungs. Any exercise that uses large muscles like those in your legs, your bottom or your chest in a repetitive and prolonged manner and makes you breathe deeper and harder, is referred to as *aerobic* exercise. So exercise such as walking, cycling, jogging, climbing stairs, playing football, rugby, rowing, tennis and even abseiling all count. Throwing darts, playing billiards and fishing (unless it's a long walk to the river bank) don't.

3 *Aerobic* means 'with air'. The air we breathe is a mixture of 79 per cent nitrogen, around 21 per cent oxygen and 0.03 per cent carbon dioxide. At rest, most people fill their lungs with about 0.4 litres of air. With exercise, this can increase tenfold to 4 litres or more. When you exercise, your working muscles need an extra supply of oxygen to break down the body's stores of glucose and fat that provide the energy that power the muscles. At rest, your body is idling at a traffic light, using the minimum amount of fuel, or oxygen. As you speed down the motorway, more fuel is delivered to power the engine, just as more oxygen is delivered to the working muscles when you exercise.

4 With regular, prolonged aerobic exercise, you will experience a 'training effect' which means that the capacity of your lungs increases so that they take in more air, even at rest. Your heart also becomes stronger so that it is able to pump out more oxygen-loaded blood with every beat. This in turn leads to a lower resting heart rate. Other training effects of regular aerobic exercise include an increase in mitochondria. These are the power cells contained within the body's muscles that generate the energy to make them contract. Aerobic activity also brings with it other metabolic changes such as an improved efficiency in dealing with body fats and sugars and converting these into energy.

5 Whichever form of physical activity or exercise you choose, there are some universal guidelines that apply every time you get moving.

- Always warm up.
- Aim to give your heart a workout by exercising aerobically for at least 20 minutes. (You may need to build up to this by starting with 10 minute bouts of aerobic activity if you are very unfit.)
- Always cool down at the end of your workout, including some stretching.

Warm up

6 Skipping the warm up of an exercise session is like trying to start your car in third gear on a frosty morning. However tempting it may be to get straight into your aerobic activity at the highest, calorie-burning level, it is never a good idea to miss your warm up. Warming up means exactly that – gradually raising your body's temperature in preparation for exercise. As your body gets warmer, hormones that dilate the blood vessels are released, enabling more blood to be transported to the working muscles and away from the internal organs. As the muscles become warmer, the individual muscle fibres become more stretchy and pliable and less likely to tear. For the body to perform efficiently, you need to give your own internal oil, called synovial fluid, a chance to lubricate the joints. As you start to move and take your muscles through their range of movement, the synovial fluid in the joints warms up and becomes less sticky, enabling the moving parts of the joints to glide smoothly over each other.

7 A thorough warm up means you're much less likely to injure yourself. The colder the weather or the ambient temperature, the longer your warm up needs to be. Also, the longer and harder your workout the longer your warm up should take.

8 Warming up need not necessarily be difficult or complicated. If you are going for a brisk walk, then you just need to start with some gentle walking and gradually increase the pace. You may like to add in some shoulder rolls to loosen the upper back and neck, and perhaps lift your knees a little higher a few times to take the knee joint through a greater range of movement. If you are about to play a demanding game of football, rugby or squash, then your coach will probably get you to perform a more thorough warm up. This will include some gentle jogging, followed by some mobilisation exercises (where you

perform gradually larger and larger movements with your arms, legs, back and neck) and, once you are warm, some gentle stretching exercises.

9 Whatever activity you take up, make sure you take time to educate yourself about the best way to perform safely and effectively. This is likely to mean that you need to understand the muscles you will be using so that you can warm them up appropriately and avoid injury or strain.

10 Warm up should last between 5 and 15 minutes, depending on the intensity of the exercise you are about to perform and your level of fitness.

8 Basic warm up routine

Raising your pulse

1 Start with some gentle walking, gradually stepping up the pace. If you are about to perform an activity that is more strenuous than walking, then start with a gentle jog. Gradually build up until you are running, without letting your breathing get out of control. You may find it useful to refer to the Rating of

Using the RPE Scale

The rating of perceived exertion scale can be useful in helping you to 'listen' to your body. Just as listening to the engine on your car can give you clues about its performance and potential problems, listening to your body will help you identify the right exercise intensity for you. Before you decide on a number, think about how you are feeling, including how hard you are breathing, how fast your heart is beating, how much you're sweating and how much your legs are aching. In studies, RPE has been shown to give an accurate reflection of how hard people are working. People who worked at around 70% of their maximum consistently describe this intensity as 'moderate', or between 4 and 6 on the scale. Seventy per cent of your maximum heart rate is the optimum level for aerobic fitness. Just remember that this is a personal scale, so your rating of perceived exertion at a particular work rate is likely to be very different to someone else's.

Perceived Exertion Scale in Section 4. Your warm up should take you to levels 3, 4 and 5 on the scale. Once you are able to sustain an RPE of 5 for 10 minutes, you are ready to move onto the main part of your workout.

2 Alternatively, if you are working out using a heart rate monitor then you need to warm up by keeping your heart rate at about 50% of its maximum for the first five minutes or so and then gradually increase to 60-70% of your maximum heart rate.

Warm-up routine

* **Start at the top and work your way down your body**
* **Breathe in deeply and then breathe out again. Relax**

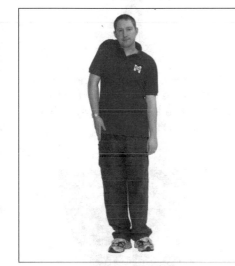

Lift your shoulders towards your ears and then down again

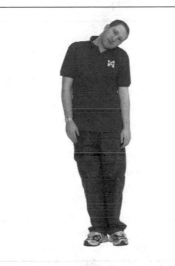

Bend the head to one side, letting your ear drop towards your shoulder and hold for 5-10 seconds. Repeat to other side

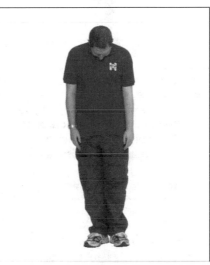

Drop your chin towards your chest to loosen your neck. Do not roll your head backwards as this compresses the vertebrae in the neck

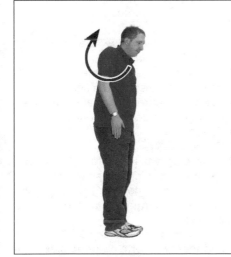

Lift your shoulders again and circle them a few times

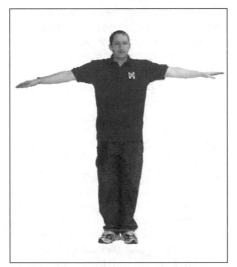

Gradually extend the arms and continue to circle your shoulders

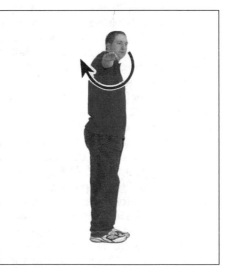

Circle the arms, keeping them slightly bent, making progressively larger and larger circles. Keep the movements controlled and avoid flinging your arms around

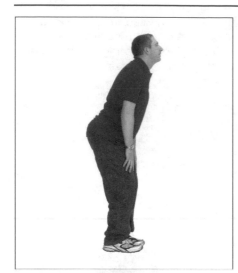

Bend your knees slightly and place your hands on your thighs. Curl the torso forwards, pulling in your stomach so the back arches. Gradually uncurl your torso, straightening the knees last of all

Place your hands on your waist and circle your hips

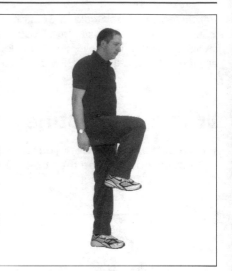

Lift one knee as high as you can and then the other, holding onto something if you are likely to lose your balance

9 Finding your training zone – working aerobically

1 Once you have warmed up, it is time to take your body into its 'training zone'. To do this, you gradually increase the intensity of your workout to a level that you can maintain for 20 minutes or more without getting out of breath. Using the RPE scale is a useful way of gauging whether you are exercising at the right pace. You can also use a simple 'talk test' to monitor how hard you are working. You should be able to carry on a conversation while you exercise. If you find this difficult, you are working too hard.

2 A more precise way of finding your training zone is to measure your heart rate or your pulse while you are exercising. You can do this by simply counting the number of beats by feeling your pulse in your wrist but you can get a more accurate measurement by using a heart rate monitor. Your training zone can be calculated once you have established your estimated maximum heart rate. To do this, you need to subtract your age from 220. So for a 40 year old man, his estimated maximum heart rate is calculated as follows:

220 – 40 = 180 bpm

3 Your training zone is between 50 per cent and 85 per cent of your estimated maximum heart rate. If you work at a rate higher than 85 per cent you will be working *anaerobically*. This means that your muscles start to rely on different forms of energy that work without oxygen. Working at high intensity (or 'anaerobically') produces a build up of lactic acid in the muscles that prevents you from exercising for very long and leaves you gasping for air. If you are very unfit, you will reach your anaerobic threshold very quickly. As you become fitter you body becomes more efficient at delivering oxygen to the working muscles enabling you to go further and faster.

4 To find your training zone, first find the lower figure by multiplying your estimated maximum heart rate by 0.50:
• *180 x 0.50 = 90 bpm*

5 Then find the upper level of your training zone:
• *180 x 0.85 = 153 bpm*

6 So, if you are a 40 year old man, your training zone is between 90 and 153 beats per minute. You should aim to keep you heart rate in this range when you are exercising. You will find that you get the most benefit from your exercise if you work at around 65% to 85% of your estimated maximum heart rate for at least 20 minutes at a time.

Training principles

Source: The Official FA Guide to Fitness for Football, *published by Hodder*

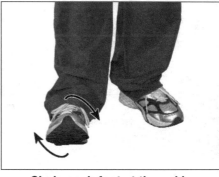

Circle each foot at the ankle

Education. See inside rear cover for further information.

7 In general terms fitness is often referred to as 'the four S's', namely:
• Stamina or cardiovascular endurance
• Strength or muscular endurance
• Suppleness or flexibility
• Speed

8 The diagram takes this theory one step further and identifies several fitness parameters and the links between them, all of which contribute to the player's performance.

9 In order to improve any or all of these components, certain principles will always apply. Adherence to these principles will ensure that the physical and physiological development of players will be optimal, whereas neglect can often result in unnecessary injury.

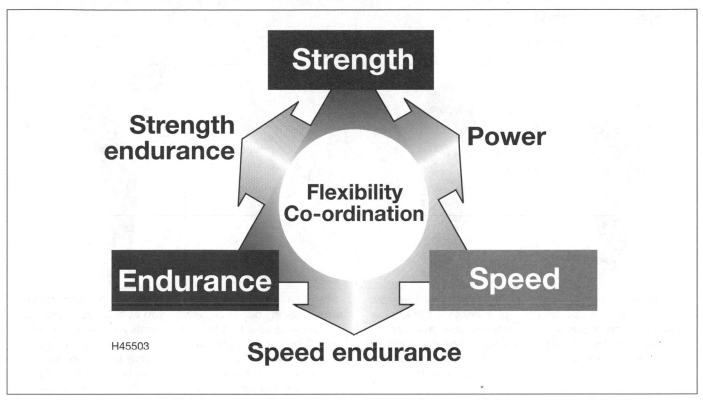

Fitness components contributing to the performance of players

Source: The Official FA Guide to Fitness for Football, *published by Hodder Education. See inside rear cover for further information.*

10 Cooling down

1 While you've been exercising, your heart has been pumping blood forcefully around the body. As the muscles in your legs contract and relax, they assist in pumping the deoxygenated blood back to the heart. If you suddenly stop exercising, the blood can pool in your lower legs leaving an insufficient supply of blood going to the brain. This can lead to dizziness and fainting and, if you are very unfit, can put undue stress on your heart. Never skip a cool down and, if you have to stop during exercise, always try to keep your feet moving to avoid blood pooling.

11 Stretching

1 Regular stretching will help keep you supple and, according to some experts, help prevent injury. Although there has been limited research into the benefits of stretching, most athletes believe that

stretching is a good idea and that it helps prevent some of the muscle soreness that can occur after a heavy workout. As you get older, your muscles and tendons being to shorten and tighten, leaving you less supple. Regular stretching won't burn calories or give you big muscles, but it will enable you to perform better and give you a greater range of movement. Stretching the muscles at the back of the thighs, the hamstrings, and the lower back is particularly beneficial in preventing the loss of flexibility that occurs with age.

How to stretch

2 NEVER stretch cold muscles. Most people find stretching after their cool down the best time, when their muscles are still warm from exercise. Stretching after a workout is also a good way to return the body to a resting state by gradually winding down and bringing the body temperature back to normal.

3 Try to stretch at least three times a week, holding each stretch for between 10 and 30 seconds. When you stretch the muscles in the back of the thighs and lower back, hold for at least 30 seconds

to develop flexibility in those areas. Do not hold any stretch if it causes you pain or if you feel pins and needles. Do not take any stretch further than is comfortable.

12 Building strength

1 However convincing those old Charles Atlas ads are, be assured that six packs and bulging biceps are not the result of weight-lifting alone. To lose fat, you need to work out aerobically. No number of sit-ups is going to get rid of your belly unless you combine them with some fat-burning exercise. But strength training can help in your efforts to shed the pounds. Muscle, as well as being heavier than fat, also uses more energy, which means that the higher your lean mass (or the more muscle you have) the higher your metabolic rate, even at rest.

2 While you burn off the bulk of your excess fat with your aerobic exercise programme, you can start to add definition to your muscles by using

Basic stretching routine

- **Start from the top and work down**

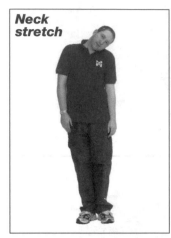

Neck stretch

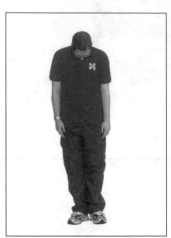

Gently let your ear drop down towards one shoulder until you feel a gentle stretch down the side of your neck. Repeat on the other side

Drop your chin towards your chest to stretch the back of your neck. Avoid taking the head backwards as this can compress the vertebrae in the neck

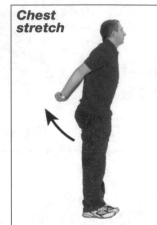

Chest stretch

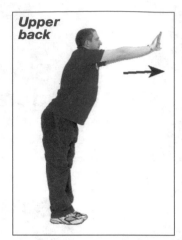

Upper back

Stand up tall and take the arms behind your back. Try to clasp your hands together and gently lift the arms away from the back. You should feel the stretch in your shoulders, chest and arms. Try not to arch your back and keep the shoulders relaxed and down

Lift your arms in front of you at shoulder height and clasp your hands together in front of you. Round the upper back and push the hands away. You should feel the stretch across your upper back, shoulders and in your arms

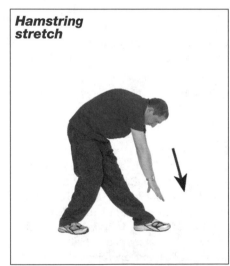

Hamstring stretch

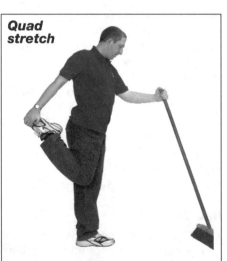

Quad stretch

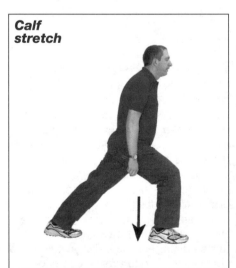

Calf stretch

You can stretch your hamstrings either standing up or sitting down on the floor. Extend one leg in front of you, keeping the other slightly bent. Reach forwards towards your toes and hold the stretch for a few seconds. Then gradually take the stretch a little further, aiming to hold it for at least 30 seconds in total

This stretches the muscles at the front of the thigh. Standing on one leg (you may need to hold onto something to steady yourself), gradually bend one leg up behind you, holding onto your foot. Keep the other leg slightly bent and avoid locking out the knee joint on the straight leg. Push the hips forward and keep the knees together

Take one leg back one step behind the body. Keeping the back leg straight, push the heel down into the ground. Keep the back foot pointing forwards. Repeat on the other leg, holding the stretch for 10 seconds

strength training and weights. Most exercise classes will use a combination of aerobic exercise and strength training, followed by some flexibility work. Similarly, if you join a gym, your instructor should give you some guidance about which pieces of apparatus will give you a balanced workout. If you are working out at home, take time to educate yourself about the best way to build strength and tone your muscles, without losing sight of the fact that any comprehensive fitness programme designed to lose weight will prioritise aerobic work. Good bookshops carry a wide range of books on the subject of weight training and strength training. The internet is also a good source of advice on how to lift weights and bulk up, if that is what you want to achieve.

Strength training top tips

- Always warm up before performing any exercise.
- Always ensure that you are performing the exercises correctly, with the proper posture in order to minimise injury.
- Start with high repetitions of low weights and build up gradually to low repetitions of higher weights.
- Incorporate strength training into two of your weekly sessions initially, always allowing rest days between training sessions.
- Seek professional guidance about weight lifting and strength training to avoid injury.

Rest periods between exercise sessions

According to the FA, the ideal weekly strength training régime should be three times a week, leaving a day to rest between bouts - for example Monday, Wednesday and Friday, resting on the other days. This allows the muscle to recover from the intense bouts of exercise so that it can work maximally at the next exercise session.

However, for those who can't commit this much time to training, please be aware that rest is a crucial factor of training and that a number of continuous days strength / endurance exercise at any one time over a short period is not desirable.

13 What's the right type of exercise?

Consider your current fitness level

1 In choosing which activity to take up, you need to consider a number of factors, not least of which is your current level of fitness. You may have once enjoyed playing in the back row at rugby (although if you've not done much exercise since, you may now look like you're more suited to prop), but remember that a demanding sport like this will require a minimum level of stamina. You will have to gradually build that fitness up, perhaps over several months, before you are able to go back to your favourite sport. If that is the case, then you can choose from a variety of activities that will gently ease you back to form. If you are very unfit, then chose exercise such as walking or cycling or join a gym where you can work at your own pace. If you are heavy, choose low-impact activities that don't put too much strain on your joints. As you become fitter and lose weight, you can move onto other, high impact activities like squash and running.

For weight loss, you need to prioritise activities that are aerobic and can be sustained for at least 20 minutes at a time. Including activities that build up your strength and will increase your muscle mass. The higher your proportion of lean muscle mass (as opposed to fat), the higher your metabolic rate will be (the rate at which your body burns calories).

Time, cost and accessibility

2 Another thing to bear in mind when choosing your activities is how easily accessible they are. To be beneficial, you need to exercise several times a week. There is no point in having abseiling as your main activity if you are only going to be able to take part once in a blue moon. Aim to build up a variety of activities that you enjoy so that you can meet the guidelines of a minimum of 30 minutes on at least five days a week. If you chose to take up or go back to football, then make sure you are complementing this with regular walking or cycling or some other activity that you can do regularly such as swimming or gym workouts.

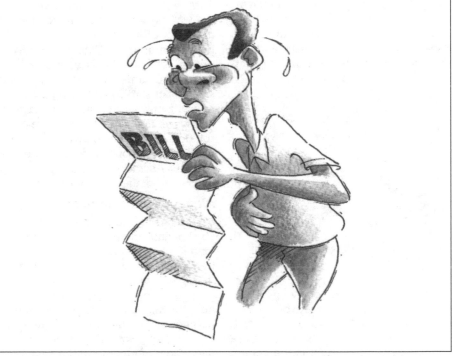

When you choose an activity, will you be able to afford the fees?

Consider the cost of the activity you are choosing, including the cost of any equipment or membership fees. Is it affordable, or will you use the cost as an excuse to give up in a few months time?

Have fun and make friends

3 Finally, chose activities that are fun. Punishing or gruelling workouts that you don't enjoy and that leave you feeling exhausted are unlikely to be sustained. Studies have shown that people who exercise with other people are more likely to stick with it than those who exercise alone. Choose sociable activities whenever possible. The social contact will also improve your mental health.

Exercising outdoors

4 You don't have to go to a gym to get fit. There is a huge gym right out there on your doorstep and it's free. Pedalling on a stationary bicycle in front of the telly may seem appealing on a cold winter's evening, but there's nothing quite like getting out into the fresh air and battling the elements. You'll have more fun, burn more calories and gain additional benefits if you take your workout outside. Humans have an instinctive need to be part of the natural world. Scientists have coined the term 'biophilia' to describe man's natural affinity with nature. Studies have shown that just being out in nature can have a positive effect on people's moods. Outdoor activities give an extra dimension to your workouts and can make them more enjoyable which means you're more likely to stick with it.

14 Walking

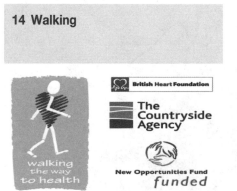

1 Walking more is probably one of the simplest ways of increasing your activity levels. Nearly everyone can do it, it requires little or no equipment and carries very little risk of injury. It is the perfect exercise for anyone who is returning to activity after a long time or following injury or illness. If you are very out of shape, then walking is the perfect way to start, and continue a fitness programme.

2 Nearly every day a new study is published extolling the virtues of walking. It has been shown to increase 'good' cholesterol (HDL) by up to 6 percent, reduce blood pressure and reduce the risk of heart disease and stroke. Experts believe that walking just a few miles per week may help prevent heart disease, diabetes, and some forms of cancer. In addition, walking has been shown to have emotional benefits such as relieving stress and helping with depression and anxiety.

How

3 Walking really is as simple as putting one foot in front of the other and has the advantage of carrying very little risk of injury, whatever your fitness level. You can increase the intensity of your walking workout by adding hills or increasing your speed. Consider joining a health walk group in your area. More information can be found on the Walking the way to Health website (see below for contact details). There are also some walking groups that are aimed specifically at disabled people.

Walk tall, pull in your gut

4 Adopting a good posture while you are walking will ensure that you get the most out of it and reduce your risk of back pain or injury. Walk tall and try to pull in your gut. Relax your shoulders and let your arms swing naturally by your side. Make sure you are using the whole of your foot when you step out. Place the heel down first and allow your weight to roll down the outside of your sole and across the ball of your foot towards the big toe. As the heel lifts, continue to push off from the ball of your foot.

Monitor your progress

5 Choose a circular route near to where you live and time yourself to find out how long it takes you to complete it. Aim to beat your time by a few seconds every time you walk. Over several weeks you should find that you get quicker and are able to walk faster and further without getting out of breath. Walk at every opportunity. Get off the bus a stop earlier, park further from the shops and use the stairs more. Add variety by seeking out walks further afield in parks or countryside. If you have a shopping mall near you, then this could be a perfect venue for walking on cold, wet days.

Count your steps

6 Consider buying or borrowing a pedometer or step-o-meter that counts the number of steps that you take each day. Experts believe that we should aim to walk 10,000 steps each day. People in this country walk on average just 4,000 steps a day. Try to increase the number of steps you take by 10 per cent each week.

Invest in a good pair of shoes

7 If walking is your main form of physical activity, you should invest in a good pair of walking shoes or walking trainers. Although you may think it is just a manufacturer's ploy, you do need to replace your shoes every 1,000 to 1,500 miles. Shoes really do wear out that quickly and, when they do, you are more likely to experience joint pain and risk injury. If you are overweight or if you start running, you will find that your shoes wear out even more quickly and no longer give your foot the support it needs. A common complaint in overweight walkers is plantar fasciitis or

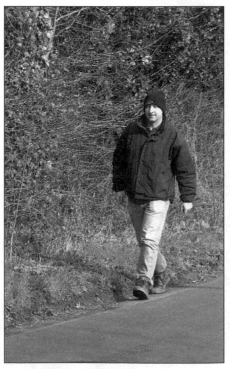

Walk tall

heel pain which can become very uncomfortable during a walk. If you experience this, check that your shoes still have enough 'spring' in them. People with flat feet, high arches or tight Achilles tendons are particularly prone to this condition. It can be alleviated by stretching the foot, but you may want to consider consulting a podiatrist who will be able to advise you and may prescribe orthotic inserts for your shoes.

Take it further

8 As you get fitter, you can start to build in short bouts of running. Try running for one minute every 5 minutes or so. Gradually increase the amount of running. Consider keeping yourself motivated by walking for a charity or set yourself a challenge by walking in a local marathon.

Pros

- *Walking is simple, free and very safe.*
- *Walking is adaptable – you can build it into your everyday life.*
- *Walking suits most levels of fitness.*
- *You don't need any special equipment or clothing.*
- *It can be made as easy or as hard as your like. Just add hills or speed up.*

Cons

- *Let's face it, it's not very macho or exciting.*
- *Unless you join a walking group it can be a little lonely.*
- *It's not going to give you Arnold Schwarzenegger muscles.*

Further information

9 If you would like to know more, look in the Contacts section at the back of the book, or contact:
Walking the way to health initiative (WHI)
Website: www.whi.org.uk
Recommended reading
'Walking for Health' Caroll and Brown

15 Cycling

1 Cycling is an excellent way to get fit. Like walking, you can build it into your everyday life by cycling to work or to the shops. It is also a low impact activity, which means that it doesn't put too much strain on your joints. The downside is that you do need to wear the right gear to be safe. Don't even think about saddling up without a helmet on your head. Even on the quietest roads you are still at risk from other road users. Too few dedicated cycle routes mean that you will often have to share the road with much faster and larger vehicles so make sure you can be seen, especially at night.

2 If your last encounter with a bike was your chopper-style BMX, you may get quite a shock when you visit your local cycle shop. There is now a huge array of bicycles to suit different types of terrain and different budgets. Seek out a good bike shop and take the advice of the salespeople in choosing the right cycle for you. They will ensure that the bike is right for your size and build and make adjustments to the riding position for you.

Cycling basics

3 Wear protective clothing. A helmet is essential, glasses are a good idea to keep dust and dirt out of your eyes and padded cycling shorts will make your life much more comfortable. Wear reflective clothing and equip your cycle with lights.

4 Position your seat correctly (your salesperson will advise you) and pedal at a smooth and easy cadence to avoid knee injury or strain. Relax your upper body when you cycle and avoid gripping the handlebars too tightly.

5 Learn the basics of cycle maintenance and carry a puncture repair kit.

6 A cycle computer will measure your speed and distance and can be useful in monitoring your progress and keeping you motivated

Further information

7 If you would like to know more, look in the Contacts section at the back of the book, or contact:
Sustrans
Website: www.sustrans.co.uk
Further reading
A range of cycling books is available from Haynes Publishing:
The Bike Book – complete bicycle maintenance.
The Mountain Bike Book.
The Racing Bike Book.
Cycle ride books for Birmingham & the Black Country, Bristol & Bath, London and Manchester.

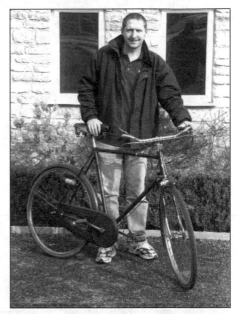

Seek out a good bike shop and take the advice of the salespeople

16 Running

1 Walking has become the new running (or jogging). If you approach any fitness professional or doctor, he is much more likely to recommend walking than running. But running still has its passionate followers and people who stick with a long term walking routine often progress to running as they find it gives them the buzz that only running can. Running is fantastic exercise and burns heaps of calories. Like walking, you can do it anywhere and it requires a minimum amount of gear. But runners also tend to experience far more injuries, particularly joint injuries, because of the relentless pounding their bodies take.

2 If you are new to exercise and fancy taking up running, then you must build up very gradually. If you are very overweight, you will need to shed those extra pounds if you are going to minimise your risk of injury from running. Start with a walking programme and gradually introduce short bouts of running, say one minute out of every five. If it hurts, stop and go back to walking. Many people find that walking gives them all the workout they need, without any of the pain that goes with pushing yourself too hard on a run.

17 Conservation work

1   Just getting out into your own garden (if you are lucky enough to have one) can be a workout in itself. Many common gardening activities such as hedge cutting, digging, mowing and weeding will give your body much of the exercise it needs (if done regularly). But there is a growing interest in the concept of 'Green Gyms'. The British Trust for Conservation Volunteers (BTCV) have been setting up conservation groups across the country (in partnership with local Primary Care Trusts and doctors' surgeries) that promise a new form of exercise; one with a tangible result at the end of it. The idea is that you go out into the countryside and carry out a variety of conservation tasks such as clearing ponds, laying hedges, building dry stone walls and fences, chopping down trees and planting new ones. There are more than 60 Green Gyms across Britain, mainly run by volunteers and operating in a variety of locations from local parks to National Trust land. The emphasis is on getting a good workout and each session starts with a warm up and ends with a cool down, including appropriate stretching exercises.

Further information

2   If you would like to know more, look in the Contacts section at the back of the book, or contact:

Green Gym
Website: www.btcv.org/greengym

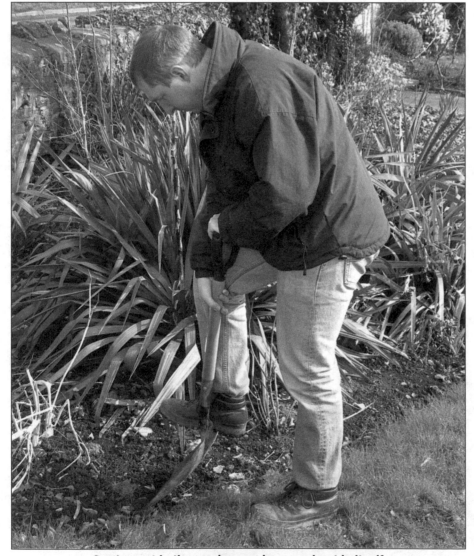
Getting out in the garden can be a workout in itself

18 Joining a gym

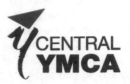

1   Joining a gym, health club or exercise class can be one of the bravest (but also the most rewarding) moves you ever make. Gyms can be daunting places and conjure up images of tanned, svelte, lycra-clad bodies doing things on pieces of equipment that look, to the uninitiated, like they belong in a medieval torture chamber. But step beyond your preconceptions and you will be pleasantly surprised to find that there are many people just like you who have found that gyms offer them all they need to get back to health and fitness.

2   There are many advantages to joining a gym, not least the fact that you will have the benefit of expert advice on hand to help you in your efforts to get back into shape. To avoid becoming one of the fifty per cent of people who quit the gym within 8 weeks of joining, you need to choose carefully. Gyms come in all shapes and sizes, with membership fees to suit most pockets. Some gyms offer very limited facilities and little professional support. The more expensive health clubs have swimming pools, jacuzzis, saunas and also offer a range of other treatments. Decide what it is you want and how much you can afford, but look for places that have fitness instructors on hand and have a range of cardiovascular training equipment (such as treadmills, cycles, stair-climbers and rowing machines) and weight training equipment.

3   Some local authority-run gyms, in conjunction with local health centres, offer subsidised schemes for heart patients and people with conditions that can benefit from exercise. Ask at your doctor's surgery whether there is an 'exercise on prescription' or exercise referral scheme near you and whether you may be eligible.

Exercise Classes

4   Don't be too quick to dismiss the idea of joining an exercise class. Although it may seem like a very hostile

environment for the average bloke, there are some classes out there that you may find surprisingly enjoyable. Check out what's on offer at your local gym, or in your local community. Look out for information from your local Adult Education centre and scour notice boards for information about classes near you. There are many classes that now cater for men, and overweight men in particular. There is a huge range on offer, from Tai Chi and Yoga, through to circuit training, stationary bikes, exercise to music classes using weights and martial arts based workouts. Joining a class is a great way to meet people and to keep motivated. Check that the instructor is qualified and is registered with the Register of Exercise Professionals (REP) before you sign up.

Personal trainers

5 If your budget can stretch to it (and it needn't cost the earth), then hiring a qualified and registered personal trainer is a smart move. If you are very out of shape or new to exercise, then you will benefit from their in-depth knowledge and ability to motivate you and help you achieve your goals. Ask for references and certificates of qualifications and whether they have public liability insurance. Make sure you like them and that you do not go on physical appearance alone. Most good trainers will understand that working out is mainly about health and not just looking the part. Look for someone who is registered with the Register of Exercise Professionals as a Personal Trainer. It is usually best to get a word of mouth recommendation, though if you don't know anyone who has a trainer, you could try calling your local gym or YMCA.

Choosing a gym

Where

6 Choose a gym that is easy for you to get to, either near your home or place of work, and make sure that the opening hours fit in with your lifestyle and work schedule. Having to drive several miles on a wet, windy night is likely to be a major deterrent to even the keenest exerciser.

Staff

7 Are they friendly and welcoming? Are they qualified to instruct? Are they REP (Register of Exercise Professionals) registered? Look for first aid qualifications as well as recognised fitness instruction qualifications such as Central YMCA qualifications or NVQ level 2. Will they give you the personal attention you need to get started and advice to help you progress through your programme? Do you like the fitness trainer whot has been assigned to you?

Costs

8 Check out exactly what is included in the membership fees and read the small print on the contract. How long do you need to sign up for? Do they offer a trial membership? Are there hidden costs such as extra charges for certain classes or parking fees? Do they offer guest passes so you can take friends along with you?

Is it clean?

9 Ask to have a thorough look around or, ideally, a trial session. Check out the showers – are they clean or are you likely to come away with more than you bargained for by picking up a nasty case of athlete's foot?

Equipment

10 Is the equipment well maintained and replaced regularly? Are there enough machines for the number of members? Visit at the times you intend to use the gym to see whether people are queuing for the machines.

Further information

11 If you would like to know more, look in the Contacts section at the back of the book, or contact:
YMCA
Tel: 020 7343 1700
Websites:
www.ymcaclub.co.uk
www.cyq.org.uk
www.ymcafit.org.uk

19 Swimming

1 Swimming is excellent aerobic activity and particularly suitable for people with joint or mobility problems. Because it is a zero-impact activity, it puts virtually no strain on the joints as the water supports your body weight. This means that it is an excellent activity for people who are overweight, although many may feel rather self-conscious about taking their clothes off in public. Just getting in and out of a swimming pool may pose a challenge for very overweight people, so check out the pool before you sign up. Does it have easy steps in and out? Are the changing rooms big enough or will you be wrestling your way in and out of a tiny cubicle?

2 If your idea of swimming is splashing around in the shallow end with the kids, then think again. To get the benefit you need from this exercise, you need to actually swim. Swimming does require a certain amount of technique and, if you haven't swum for a while, or if you are new to swimming, it may be a good idea to book a few private lessons to get you started. Alternatively, look out for water aerobics classes that provide excellent exercise for all shapes and sizes.

20 Choosing sport

SPORT ENGLAND

Why choose sport?

1 Cast your eyes around the terraces of your local football ground. What do you see? Lots of overweight, HGV models just like yourself, enjoying the game with their kids, knocking back calorie-laden hot dogs and drinks. It is ironic that many of the people who love watching sport are the very people who have the most to gain from *participating*. But making the transition from the couch to the pitch may be something you have never considered. If you thought that watching your favourite team win was thrilling, just try getting out there and doing it yourself. Because so many of the HGV models have an innate interest in sport, you are already at an advantage when it comes to playing it. You know the rules, the statistics, the jargon. You just need to work on the body to go with it. Even though you may not be in the peak of fitness, this does not mean that you cannot find a sport that you can do.

2 Sport has all the ingredients that you need to get fitter and healthier. It's fun, it's sociable, it's exciting and, thanks to massive investment by organisations such as Sport England, it is becoming much more accessible to all. Taking part in sport can get you involved with your local community. Your knowledge of a particular sport may mean that you are able to help with coaching or volunteer to organise sporting events for your local teams. Just getting out and being active will help to improve your health, even if you are not playing or competing.

3 Although some sports require a minimum level of fitness in order to take part, there are many that are particularly suitable for heavier or unfit people. Many clubs now also offer opportunities for less fit people to take part through beginners' teams or specialised groups.

Which sport?

4 Try to choose a sport that will give you an aerobic workout, but not tax you so much that you are unable to sustain it for more than a few minutes. Some sports require only very low levels of fitness, such as croquet or bowls. These types of sport are unlikely to improve your fitness much or help you lose weight, but getting out in the fresh air and meeting people has been shown to be good for your health too. If you do choose a 'low fitness' sport, try to supplement the physical activity you do with walking or cycling more.

5 When choosing which sport to take up, consider the following factors:

Fitness level

6 Some sports are more physically demanding than others. Choose less demanding sports such as badminton or golf that can be easily adapted to your own pace. As your fitness improves, you can start to consider sports such as football or squash. Although some sports are very demanding at a competitive level, many clubs offer opportunities for fun and 'friendly' games. Don't dismiss soccer just because you can't keep up with the 'A' team, there may be other teams within the club more suited to your current level of fitness. Seek out people with a similar level of fitness to your own to compete against.

Skill level

7 Although some sports (such as the martial art of Aikido) require only a low level of fitness, they may involve a high level of skill and take many months or years to perfect. Skating (either in-line or on ice) may be an excellent way to get fit, but can you cope with the indignity of the falls (or the pain of the bruises) that go with learning?

Accessibility

8 How close is the club/the facility to where you live or work? Is it easy to get to? What are the opening hours and when do the team meet?

Cost

9 How much will the membership fees cost? What equipment do you need? Can you hire it until you know it is what you want to do? Do you need insurance? (some extreme sports may not be covered by your current insurance policy).

10 Below is a list of some sports you may wish to consider. Although many sports require a high level of fitness and skill at a competitive level, many clubs now offer beginners' opportunities and introduction programmes for less fit people. Many sports are adaptable to your level of fitness simply by choosing to compete against people of a similar fitness and skill level to yourself.

Further information

11 If you would like to know more, look in the Contacts section at the back of the book, or contact:

Sport England
Website: www.sportengland.org.uk
Sport near you?
Website: www.activeplaces.com

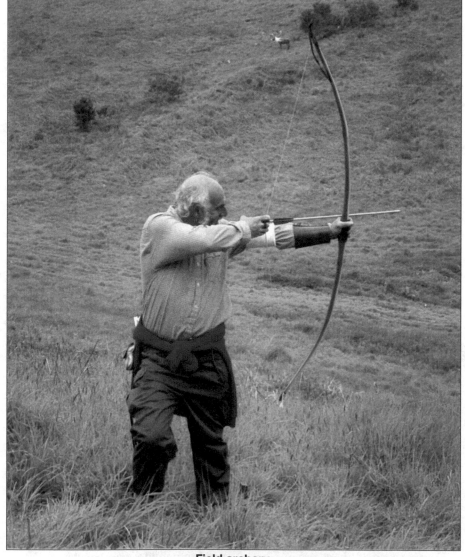

Field archery
Photo courtesy Richard Head Longbows (www.english-longbow.co.uk)

Sport	Minimum Fitness required	Minimum Skill required	Contact
Aikido	Low	High	www.aikido-uk.org
Archery	Low	Medium to High	www.gnas.org
Baseball	Low	Low	Baseball Softball UK 020 7453 7055
Badminton	Low to Medium	Low to Medium	www.baofe.co.uk
Basketball	High	High	www.hoops.co.uk
Cricket	Low to Medium	Medium	www.play-cricket.com
Fencing	Medium	Medium to High	www.britishfencing.com
Field sports	Low to Medium	Medium to High	www.ukathletics.org
Football	Low to High	Medium	www.the-FA.org
Golf	Low to Medium	Medium	www.englishgolfunion.org
Karate	Low to Medium	Medium	www.ekgb.org.uk
Mountain Biking	Medium	Medium	www.bcf.uk.com/www.sustrans.org.uk
Racquetball	Low to Medium	Low to Medium	www.racquetworld.com
Rowing	Medium to High	Medium	www.ara-rowing.org
Table Tennis	Low to Medium	Medium	English Table Tennis Association 01494 722525
Tennis	Low to Medium	Medium to High	www.tennis.com
Volleyball	Low to Medium	Low to Medium	www.volleyballengland.org
Water Polo	High	Medium to High	www.nwpl.co.uk
Wrestling	Medium to High	Medium to High	www.britishwrestling.org

Compiled by Kate Heighway: www.medicdirectsport.com

21 Getting your head round it

1 It is a fact that fifty percent of people who start on an exercise programme quit within 8 weeks. You may even be one of those people. You've tried it before, you've made the resolutions, bought the exercise cycle and joined the gym only to find that a few months on you're back to where you were. Or worse, even piled on more weight that when you started. You are not alone, but that does not mean that you cannot be successful. Every year there are thousands of people who do change their lives through exercise and for whom exercise does become a habit. To guarantee success, you need to plan your attack, find an activity you enjoy, set yourself some realistic goals, track your progress and reward your successes.

Visualise it

2 Keep an image in your mind of how it will feel when you've lost your weight, you're fitter and you're enjoying all the things that being overweight prevents you from doing. When your motivation starts to flag, conjure up that image in your mind to keep you focused.

Plan your attack

3 Have a good look at your current lifestyle. How do you spend your time? Where could you fit physical activity into your life? What exercise or physical activity would you enjoy?

4 The most commonly used excuse for not exercising is lack of time. Ironically, we have more leisure time now than at any point in our civilised history and yet we are not using it wisely. Watching your favourite soap every night may be your idea of unwinding, but wouldn't that time be better spent investing in your health? Perhaps you could combine the two by exercising in front of the TV? If spending time with your family is a priority, then why not choose to spend time doing active things like going to the park or

swimming or even just going for a walk? Many very busy successful people find time to exercise because they know that it actually buys them *more* time. Being fitter will give you more energy to do everyday tasks, help you sleep better so that you need less of it and improve your quality of life and health so that less of your time is wasted being ill.

- *Choose activities that you enjoy.*
- *Exercise with a partner or friend whenever possible.*
- *Choose activities that are close to your home or workplace.*

Employers are now beginning to realise that a fit workforce means less absenteeism and higher productivity. For information on how to persuade your employer to free up more time for physical activity contact:
Workplace Health Initiative
Website: www.bhf.org.uk

Setting goals
Make it personal

5 Set yourself goals that are personal to you. Getting your blood pressure down may be your doctor's idea of a goal, but is it likely to keep you motivated? Being able to fit into an old pair of jeans or keeping up with your children on a bike ride may be more relevant to you than medical statistics and more likely to keep you on track.

Write it down

6 Just writing down your goals will help to make them a reality and keeping a log of your progress will provide the extra motivation you need. Make sure your goals are specific and achievable.

Activity log

Week number . . . .

Weekly goal . . . . eg, Walk for 20 minutes every day

Day	Time spent	Type of activity	Intensity	Comments
Monday	50 minutes	Walking (20 mins) Gardening (30 mins)	60% Maximum Heart Rate (or 'Moderate')	Felt OK. Slight pain in right foot
Tuesday	50 minutes	Played ball with kids	Hard!	Fun – didn't feel like exercise

Set short, medium and long-term goals

7 Your long term goal may be to lose 3 stone and run the local 10K race, but that goal could be months or years away and you are likely to lose your motivation long before you achieve it. Setting yourself interim or short-term goals will ensure that you get a sense of achievement every week or every time you exercise.

Multiple goals

8 Set yourself multiple goals (or back-up goals). One of your goals may be to lose 2 pounds a week but the other could be to decrease your set walk route time by 30 seconds every week or to walk for five minutes longer every week. Having multiple goals means that, even if you have a week when you don't lose any weight, you can still get a sense of achievement from having completed the amount of exercise you set out to do. Pedometers are excellent for measuring and tracking your progress. The thought of trying to walk 10,000 steps a day may be quite daunting, but increasing the number of steps you do by a set percentage each week will keep you motivated.

Top tips to keep you on track
Put it in the diary

9 Mark your exercise sessions in your diary and block out the time weeks in advance.

Exercise with a friend

10 Studies have shown that people who exercise with their partner or friend are much more likely to stick with it.

11 Even if you really don't feel like your usual workout, go anyway, but make it easier.

12 You may have had a heavy night and the last thing you feel like doing is a gruelling gym workout. Go for a walk instead. Exercise is habit-forming and, unlike smoking, one that is all too easy to break.

Variety is the spice of life

13 Vary your workouts. If you walk, chose a different route or do the same route the other way round. Try cycling or swimming or explore further afield and try adventure sports like canoeing (or canoodling!) or mountain biking.

Pay in advance

14 For some people, there is nothing quite like a little financial incentive to keep you going. Forking out for those membership fees or buying a block booking of gym sessions can be a powerful motivator.

Be prepared

15 Get your kit ready the night before your workout. If your enthusiasm starts to wane, then investing in a new pair of trainers or a new bit of kit can kick start you back into action.

Record progress and measure improvement

16 Keep an exercise diary or log and measure your progress every six weeks for fitness tests you can do at home or in the gym.

Goal sheet

Long term goal	eg, Climb Snowdon, lose 3 stone
Back-up long term goals	eg, Fit into my old suit
Short term goals	eg, Cycle or walk to work at least 4 times a week
Weekly goals	eg, Cycle to work twice this week
Daily goals	eg, Walk up the stairs instead of using the escalator on my way to work

Progress report

Date	Distance walked and time	Exercise heart rate	Resting heart rate	Weight	Waist to hip ratio
12.01.05	2 miles, 32 minutes	min 90, max 167 bpm	73 bpm	102 kg	1.0
12.03.05	4 miles, 59 minutes	min 101, max 156 bpm	67 bpm	98 kg	0.96

Reward your successes and achievements

17 When you reach your goals, be they short or long-term, reward yourself with something you enjoy (but not food!). Buy yourself a CD or tickets to the cinema or football match. Go out for a drink with your mates (just the one though, or you'll undo all your hard work).

22 Injuries and how to prevent them

1 If you are unused to exercise, then you may well experience a certain amount of discomfort when you start doing any meaningful physical activity. Let's face it, if you'd left your car parked up for this long in a garage without giving it the odd service or turning over the engine once in a while, you'd be amazed if it ran smoothly at the first turn of the key. You are bound to experience the odd ache or pain after your first few bouts of exercise, but you need to be able to recognise the difference between 'good' and 'bad' pain.

2 Most common injuries associated with exercise can be avoided with careful preparation and by knowing how to recognise when you may be at risk. Before you start exercising it is important to make sure that you are fit and well enough to do so. Complete the questionnaire in Section 4 and consult your doctor if you answer 'yes' to any of the questions or if you are over 45 and are unused to exercise.

3 Being overweight will put you at greater risk from injury, so it is vital that you take necessary precautions to ensure that you don't hurt yourself. If you suffer from a condition such as diabetes, or high blood pressure, or you suffer from joint pain, then you may need to take extra care when exercising, but your doctor should be able to advise you on your specific condition.

4 Pain is your body's warning light and, as everyone knows, warning lights should not be ignored. It is your body's way of telling you that you are asking it to do something that may cause it damage. Generally speaking, a dull, achy pain that you feel throughout an entire muscle is a sign that it has been worked beyond its usual load but is nothing to worry about. This type of pain usually subsides within a day or so and is associated with fatigue. It can be prevented or alleviated by following a proper warm up and cool down and by building up gradually when you exercise.

5 If a pain is sharp and concentrated on a particular part of the body, or if it hurts when you do particular movements, then this is a sign of a specific injury and should be treated. Ignore this type of pain at your peril, as it usually requires rest and treatment to improve. Without treatment, the injury could be made worse and require an extended period of rest which will prevent you from continuing with your exercise programme.

Top tips for avoiding injury

Warning lights

6 Listen to your body and learn to recognise the difference between discomfort and pain.

Move up through the gears one by one

7 Warm up, cool down and build up gradually.

Distribution of training and match injuries throughout the season

Source: FA Injury Audit (2001), Hawkins (2001)

As you can see from the graph, the greatest percentage of football injuries happen in July. This is when players return to training from the 'close season'. In most cases these injuries will happen because training programmes are designed to expect too much, too soon.

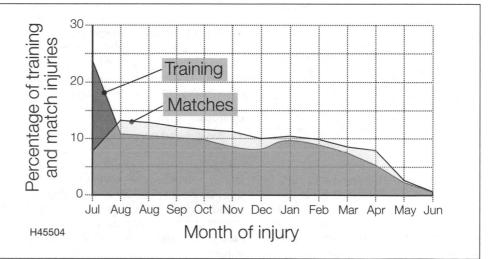

H45504

Know your performance limits

8 Work at YOUR OWN PACE and do not be tempted to compete with others who may be much fitter than yourself.

Know the highway code

9 Learn to perform the exercise correctly and take care when lifting weights or starting a new sport.

Don't rag it around

10 Limit the amount of time you spend on a new activity or exercise to 20 minutes at a time AT THE MOST. If the activity is particularly strenuous, do no more than 5 minute bouts and alternate with other muscle groups.

Check fuel before you start

11 Drink plenty of water before and during exercise to avoid dehydration. If you are diabetic, ensure that you plan when you eat or when you need your insulin injections around your exercise session. Diabetics should always carry glucose in liquid or tablet form.

Common exercise injuries

Muscle strain

12 This usually occurs when you have over-stretched a muscle or torn part of the tendon that attaches the muscle to the bone. Stop the activity and treat with the RICE method. Most muscle strain can be avoided with proper warm up and gradually building up the activity.

Sprain

13 A sprain usually refers to a torn or over-stretched ligament and occurs most commonly in the ankle as a result of an accident such as falling off a curb. The area will usually swell up and require treatment. In the first instance, follow the RICE treatment.

Shin splints

14 This is a term used to describe pain in the lower leg, below the knee. This type of pain usually comes on slowly and subsides with rest. It is usually the result of stepping up the pace too quickly or ill-fitting shoes. It should subside with rest and be alleviated by a longer warm up.

Chafing

15 This is very common and can be extremely uncomfortable. It is caused by clothing (or skin) repeatedly rubbing against sweaty skin. Untreated, it can put you out of action for several days. Prevention is the best cure, so at the first

sign of irritation, apply talcum powder or petroleum jelly to the affected area to reduce the friction

Plantar fasciitis (heel pain)

16 This is a common injury of the foot, particularly among overweight people or as a result of wearing shoes that have too little support or 'spring' left in them. The plantar fascia is a band of fibres that extend from the heel to the base of the toes. Because of its position and the amount of weight that it bears, it can take quite a battering during exercise and can become inflamed, leading to pain deep in the heel pad. People with flat feet or high arches are particularly prone to this condition. Experiment with different types of trainers, or heel or shoe inserts and apply the RICE principle when the pain is acute. Stretch the muscles of the foot and the calf regularly to help prevent some of the pain.

Knee pain

17 Knee pain is usually associated with overdoing things or choosing inappropriate exercise for your body type and fitness level. The more weight you carry, the more your knees will be at risk, particularly from high impact activities or exercise that involves lots of twisting and turning. Choose low-impact activities such as walking and cycling and consult your doctor if the pain persists or caused by a specific activity.

Back pain

18 Most cases of back pain disappear within four weeks without any treatment at all. Contrary to popular belief, the worst thing you can do is to rest completely. This will only weaken the muscles of the back. Choose low-impact activities such as walking and keep moving. Most back pain is improved with regular exercise, particularly back pain associated with being overweight.

Blisters

19 Blisters and sores are very common among new exercisers and should be treated as soon as possible to prevent infection. Diabetics are particularly at risk due to poor circulation and loss of sensation in the feet. It is important that they check their feet regularly for blisters and sores and wear properly fitting shoes.

The RICE principle

The RICE principle refers to a common way of treating sports injuries. RICE stands for Rest, Ice, Compression and Elevation. If used at the first sign of injury, it will usually alleviate symptoms within 48 hours. If an injury persists, consult your doctor.
- Rest – Stop the activity you are doing and rest the muscle that hurts.
- Ice – Apply an ice pack, cold compress or just a bag of frozen peas to the affected area.
- Compression – Apply pressure to the area by wrapping a bandage tightly around it.
- Elevation – Keep the affected limb elevated by raising it onto a chair or on some pillows. This will help fluid and waste products drain from the area and reduce swelling.

23 Fuel for exercise

1 Put the wrong fuel in your tank and you'll end up with an under-performing engine. Eat healthily, on a daily basis, and your body will be able to respond to the demands you make of it when you exercise. Any regular exerciser will vouch for the fact that their performance is seriously affected after an evening on the beer. Excessive drinking can lead to weight gain, but it can also seriously affect your resolve when it comes to dieting and exercise. If you haven't given up smoking already, then doing so as you start a new exercise regime will mean you are more likely to succeed and mean that you're not gasping for air every time you step up the pace.

2 Some foods are better than others for exercisers. Choose carbohydrate-rich foods, but avoid eating a large meal at least two hours before your exercise session. During exercise, the blood is diverted from your digestive system to your working muscles. Eating a large meal just before you exercise may leave you feeling sluggish and unwell. A small pre-exercise snack, 30 minutes before exercise, should provide you with all the energy you need. Keep away from sugary and high fat foods. The following are all excellent choices:

• *Fruit.*
• *A small sandwich.*
• *Bananas.*
• *Raisins.*
• *Fruit juice.*

It takes a nine mile walk to burn off the calories in a cheeseburger meal with chips and a milkshake.

Keep the water topped up

3   Keeping the body hydrated during exercise is crucial. Don't wait until you are thirsty to drink, as thirst is a sign that the body has already become dehydrated. Drink at least one glass of water before your workout and continue sipping every 10 minutes or so during exercise. Your body needs at least 4 pints of water a day. If you exercise, particularly in hot conditions, then you will need at least twice that amount. During exercise, your body produces waste products as a result of converting fat and protein into energy. As well as keeping you cool and hydrated, water flushes out these waste products from your body. Signs of poor hydration include dizziness, nausea, tiredness and headaches. You can tell from the colour of your pee if you are drinking enough water; clear or light yellow pee is sign of good hydration.

24 Exercising with a disability

1   Recent legislation in the UK, through the Disability Discrimination Act, has meant that many more opportunities have opened up for disabled people wanting to be physically active. The paralympic movement has spawned a new generation of disabled sportsmen and women and inspired many (who thought their exercising days were over) to take up new activities.

2   Many gyms now provide a range of equipment specifically designed for the disabled such as recumbent cycles and upper body ergometers. Your local authority should be able to advise you what is available in your area. Many forms of exercise and sport can be adapted for the disabled so it is a good idea to contact any organisations involved to see what they can provide for you. Unfortunately there is still a shortage of trained professionals to help and advise individuals as to the best form of physical activity for them, but access to facilities is improving. Many popular walks and footpaths have been opened up for wheelchair users and there are several organisations offering walks with 'buddy' systems for the visually impaired.

3   Sport England has recently funded a countrywide initiative called Inclusive Fitness, funding 150 different Local Authority, Education and YMCA sites across the country to provide facilities for disabled exercisers. All will have trained and qualified staff who can work with disabled people.

Further information

4   If you would like to know more, look in the Contacts section at the back of the book, or contact:
Walking the way to health initiative (WHI)
Website: www.whi.org.uk
Inclusive Fitness Initiative
Website: www.inclusivefitness.org.uk

25 Accessories – Gizmos and Gadgets to help you get fit

1   Every week a new fitness gadget appears on the shopping channel promising you firmer abs, tighter thighs or a chest like Tarzan's. The majority of them are a complete waste of money and, before you know it, will end up in the loft along with all those useless kitchen gadgets. But there are a few gadgets, such as heart rate monitors and pedometers that are worthwhile and can really help to keep you on track and motivated.

2   Before you invest in large pieces of fitness equipment such as rowing machines, static cycles and treadmills, be confident that you will get your money's worth and that they won't end up as clothes horses in the corner of the bedroom. Always check the manufacturer's guidelines; some machines are only suitable for people less than 100 kgs in weight.

Heart Rate Monitor

3   Apart from a good pair of trainers, the next best piece of kit to buy is a heart rate monitor. Your heart rate directly reflects how hard you are working and a heart rate monitor is an excellent way of monitoring your exercise intensity. Heart rate monitors are a great tool for beginners who may be a little wary of how their body responds to exercise and they provide reassurance that you are working at the correct intensity. Heart rate monitors can also give you something tangible to focus on when you are exercising and give you a benchmark to work to. The best ones come in two parts: a chest strap containing electrodes and a watch that picks up a signal from the strap. Make sure that the strap is large enough to fit comfortably around your chest and that the electrodes can be comfortably positioned and still pick up the electrical impulses from your heart. Prices range from £30 to £300 for a version that stores your data and can be downloaded onto a computer for home analysis. Many gym machines are now compatible with heart rate monitors and will pick up the information from your chest strap and display it without the need for the watch.

Pedometers

4   A pedometer (or step-o-meter) is a gadget that clips to your belt and counts the number of steps you take. Every time you swing your leg forward a bearing in the device moves and clicks the counter on. They can also be programmed with your stride length to track distance and some provide an estimate of calories burned. Experts say that we should aim to walk 10,000 steps every day. The average person in this country manages about half that amount. By gradually increasing the number of steps that you take by 5 to 10 per cent each week, you will soon get into the walking habit and improve your health. Most pedometers keep a record of your performance over several days so you can monitor improvements and track progress. Pedometers are cheap, motivating and give lots of information in an

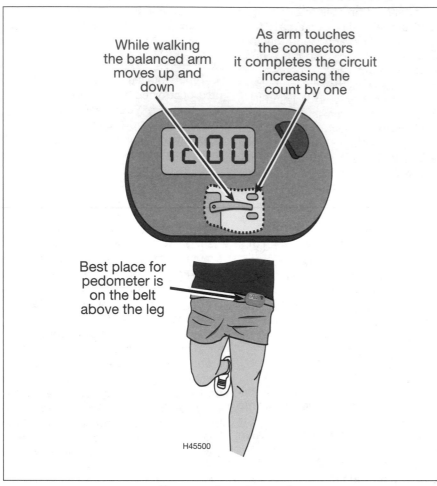

While walking the balanced arm moves up and down

As arm touches the connectors it completes the circuit increasing the count by one

Best place for pedometer is on the belt above the leg

H45500

How a pedometer works

uncomplicated package. Prices range from just a few pounds to £30. Some doctors' surgeries will loan you a pedometer and provide advice on setting it up. Some of the newer models on the market don 't need to be clipped to your belt, but can be slipped into a front pocket instead.

BP Cuffs

5 Being overweight is frequently associated with high blood pressure which is associated with a higher risk of heart disease and stroke. Many people find monitoring their blood pressure on a daily basis gives them a more accurate reflection of their condition than waiting several months between doctor's visits. As you lose weight and your fitness improves, you should see a drop in your blood pressure after a few months. Manufacturers have now brought out a whole range of blood pressure monitoring devices for use in the home. Most are easy to use and give reliable readings. Some monitors have a cuff that is worn on the upper arm and is attached to a display unit via a tube. Others are just worn around the wrist. Prices range from £50 to £200 for a unit that can transfer the data to your computer.

6 When you buy a blood pressure kit, ensure that the cuff size is correct for your arm. It is advisable to get a doctor

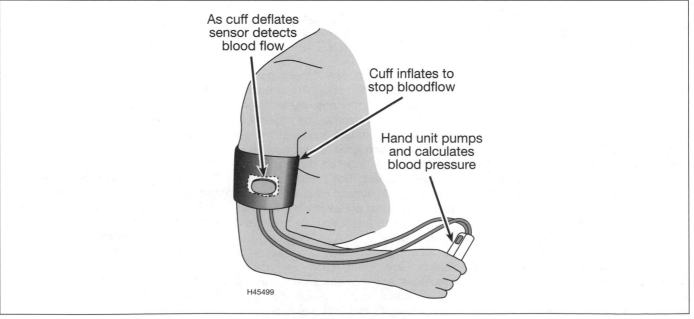

As cuff deflates sensor detects blood flow

Cuff inflates to stop bloodflow

Hand unit pumps and calculates blood pressure

H45499

BP cuff for home use

or pharmacist to measure your arm and give you a recommendation as to which cuff would be best suited to your size. Taking a measurement using a cuff that is either too big or too small will only result in an inaccurate reading which will be of no use whatsoever.

Scales

7 Look for scales that tell the whole story. There are several devices on the market that monitor your fat percentage as well as your weight. Knowing your body composition is a much more useful way of monitoring your progress. As you start to exercise, you often build more muscle (which is heavier than fat) and this may lead you to believe that you are not losing at the rate you had hoped. Knowing your fat percentage and seeing that drop will provide you with the reassurance you need that you are on track. Accuracy can be an issue with scales and body fat monitoring devices, particularly as both weight and body fat can fluctuate dramatically over a few days or even within the same day. Try to weigh yourself at the same time of day, no more than once a week.

Further information

8 If you would like to know more, look in the Contacts section at the back of the book, or contact:
Websites:
www.fitandfatinc.com
www.heartzone.com

It's never too early or too late to start being physically active, but it is always too early to stop.
Vuori, 1996

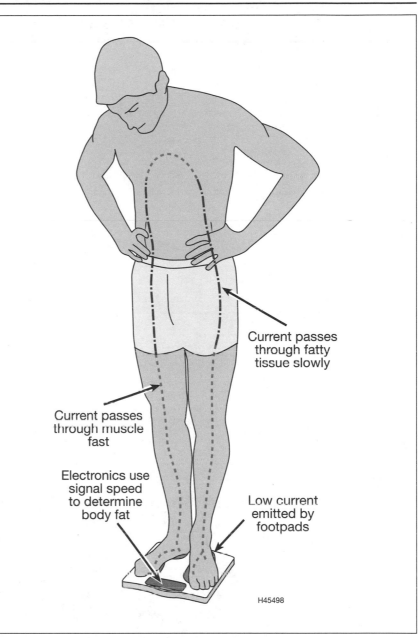

Current passes through fatty tissue slowly

Current passes through muscle fast

Electronics use signal speed to determine body fat

Low current emitted by footpads

H45498

Operating principle of body fat monitor

Chapter 4
Nutrition, water and weight control

Contents

1 Strange but true

> On average, we eat 27,215 kg (60,000 lb) of food during our life. That's equivalent to chomping our way through six elephants* or 25 rhinos.
>
> * http://www.guinnessworldrecords.com/content_pages/record.asp?recordid=48481.

Records

1 According to *The Guinness Book of Records*, the American Jon Brower Minnoch (1941–83) holds the record for being the world's heaviest person. In 1963, the 6 foot 1 inch (185 cm) Minnoch weighed 178 kg (28 stone). By 1976, he tipped the scales at 442 kg (69 stone 9 lb). In March 1978, doctors at the University Hospital, Seattle, estimated that Minnoch weighed more than 635 kg (100 stone). But getting Minnoch there wasn't easy. A dozen firemen needed to resort to an improvised stretcher and a ferry-boat. The hospital lashed two beds together to support Minnoch's bulk and it took 13 people to turn him over[1].

2 Minnoch also holds the record for the greatest weight loss. After two years on a diet of 1200 calories per day, his weight fell to 216 kg (34 stone). But by the time Minnoch died in 1983,

his weight had crept up to 362 kg (57 stone)[2].

3 Despite his immense size, Minnoch doesn't hold the record for the world's biggest chest. Robert Earl Hughes, born in 1926 in Illinois, holds that record with a button-popping 3.15 m (10 ft 4 in), according to *The Guinness Books of Records*. Hughes weighed 484 kg (1067 lb) when he died in 1958. Hughes wasn't greedy. He produced very low levels of thyroxin – a hormone that helps convert food to energy[3]. So the food he ate was put on as fat instead.

The myths

4 There is no truth in the myth that overweight men have a slow metabolism. Scientists haven't found any evidence that obese people have the extraordinarily low metabolic rates needed to account for their excess fat[4]. There is no truth in the myth that you can't do anything because the obesity is all in your genes. Your DNA controls only 25% to 40% of your body mass[5]. So between 60% and 75% – probably more – is under your control. You need to lose just 10% to gain some marked health benefits. The dramatic increase in obesity over recent years can't be due to genetic changes: it happened too quickly[6]. And there's probably no truth in the fact that you're overweight because of your hormones. Hormonal problems are uncommon and tend to result in gains of just 5 to 10 kg[7]. In any case, your doctor can easily rule these out.

References

[1] http://www.guinnessworldrecords.com/content_pages/record.asp?recordid=48383.
[2] http://www.guinnessworldrecords.com/content_pages/record.asp?recordid=48383.
[3] http://www.guinnessworldrecords.com/content_pages/record.asp?recordid=48481.
[4] Chambers R and Wakley G Obesity and Overweight Matters in Primary Care Radcliffe Medical Press 2002 Oxford p9.
[5] Mann J and Truswell AS Essentials of human nutrition 2nd edition Oxford University Press 2002 p277.
[6] Chambers R and Wakley G Obesity and Overweight Matters in Primary Care Radcliffe Medical Press 2002 Oxford p10.
[7] Mann J and Truswell AS Essentials of human nutrition 2nd edition Oxford University Press 2002 p279.

> A man who burns off 2200 kcal a day produces as much heat as a 100 watt electric light bulb left on for the same time. The bulb is smaller and the heat loss concentrated over a smaller area. That's why the bulb feels hot and you don't*.
>
> * Wiseman G Nutrition & Health Taylor & Francis 2002 p4.

2 History of men and weight

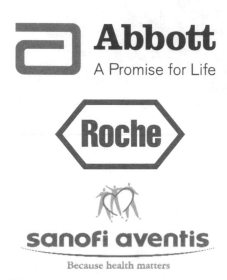

The obesity epidemic

1 We're rapidly turning into a nation of couch potatoes – more interested in watching sport than taking part. In the 1960s, the average person watched 13 hours of TV a week. We now watch, on average, more than 26 hours each week[1]. To make matters worse, many more of us now have sedentary, desk-bound jobs than in our father's generation. Our homes and garages are packed with labour saving devices. And we sometimes take the car for distances that our parents wouldn't think twice about walking. Indeed, 50 years ago, British adults burnt off the same amount of energy each week as a runner in a marathon. Today only a third of men meet the current guidelines for physical activity. This means taking moderate or vigorous activity for at least 30 minutes on five or more days a week[2].

Most overweight and obese people tend to believe that they eat about a third less food than they really do. In particular, overweight people tend to forget all the snacks that they eat*. They forget the biscuits with coffee, the crisps down the pub and the packet of chips on the way home.

* Chambers R and Wakley G Obesity and Overweight Matters in Primary Care Radcliffe Medical Press 2002 Oxford p57.

2 Unfortunately, you have to work hard to burn the calories off. Driving a car for an hour burns off just 80 kcal, that's about the same as a slice of bread. To burn off the pint-and-a-half you had at lunchtime (260 kcal) you need to walk 5 km in an hour. To lose a couple of chocolate bars (600 kcal) you'd need to run 9 km in an hour. And to get rid of your mum's roast dinner and sponge pudding (1440 kcal) you have to exercise as hard as a competitive cross-country skier for an hour[3].

3 Provided you burn the calories off you won't gain weight. But you store any extra as fat. Some researchers suggest that we consume fewer calories today than a generation ago. According to this theory, the decline in physical activity accounts for most of the increase in obesity. But data collected in the 1970s was based on the calories in the food and drink people consumed at home. The study excluded food eaten at work, in snack bars and in restaurants. It also excluded alcoholic drinks. Today, we eat out more often (and portions are often bigger[4]), consume more snacks and drink more alcohol than our parents. So it seems that eating too much as well as the decline in physical activity caused the obesity epidemic[5].

In some cultures, being fat is valued – and is even a life saver. For example, life on the isolated pacific island of Nauru is traditionally hard. The inhabitants scraped a living from agriculture and fishing, but the soil is poor and droughts common, so they frequently starved. Being fat allowed them to survive the famines, so the islanders admired big, fat people; Nauruan girls even went on diets to fatten them. Since the island moved to a more western lifestyle, rates of type II diabetes rocketed*. This ability to survive famine is probably why the genes for 'fatness' didn't die out over the course of human evolution.

* Diamond J The double puzzle of diabetes Nature 2003;423:600.

Why and when should I see my GP?

4 Obesity causes or contributes to a wide variety of diseases. Just about the only good news to come from the obesity epidemic is that doctors and the government now take excess weight more seriously than before. They're determined to help us lose weight and tackle the leading causes of ill health in the UK, such as strokes, cancers and heart disease. Indeed, the government noted in a recent white paper: "The rapid increase in child and adult obesity over the past decade is storing up very serious health problems for the future if it is not addressed effectively now." Fortunately, doctors can use a growing

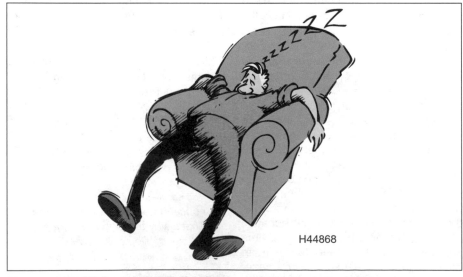

H44868

We're rapidly turning into a nation of couch potatoes

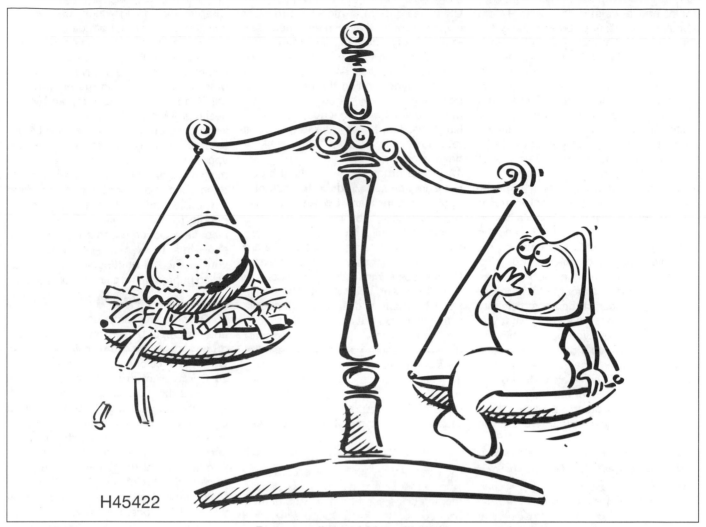

H45422

Do you really want fries with that?

number of approaches to help you lose weight. We will look at some of these later.

5 When should you see your GP? The first step is to determine if you are overweight. Your weight itself doesn't accurately reflect the risk that you'll suffer from the ill-effects of being overweight. If I'm 6 foot 4 and 175 pounds, my weight is in the healthy range. If I'm 5 foot 9 and the same weight, I'm overweight. So doctors tend to use the body mass index (BMI). This takes your height into account. A BMI of between 18.5 and 24.9 is healthy[6].

6 You can easily work out your BMI using a calculator or one of the on-line sites[7]. The BMI is your weight in kilograms divided by your height in metres squared (multiplied by itself). So Derek is 6 foot and 12 stone – that's

1.83 metres and 76.2 kg. So his BMI is: 76.2 / (1.83 x 1.83) = 22.7. A BMI between 25 and 29.9 means you're overweight. Anything over 30 is obese. If you top 40, you are severely or morbidly overweight[8] and need to see your doctor urgently. (See Chapter 5 for more on BMI.)

> *There are no marked regional differences in the prevalence of obesity in the UK when the effects of age, social class and smoking habit are allowed for.*

7 But there are a couple of problems. The BMI can't tell the difference between fat and muscle. And the BMI doesn't take account of the way fat is spread around your body[9]. So a very muscular man – a hod carrier or body builder, for

example – may have a high BMI but very little fat.

8 On the other hand, some men may not be obese, but carry a large 'beer belly'. This abdominal or central obesity indicates an accumulation of visceral fat and is particularly dangerous – and much more of a risk to your health than the fat under your skin. Each of the fat cells acts like a tiny factory pumping out chemicals that travel in the blood to other parts of your body. When they reach some parts of the body – the pancreas that produces insulin, for example – the signals can cause the organ to go wrong. That's one reason why excess fat is linked to type II diabetes and metabolic syndrome (see Section 3) which doctors now recognise is a particular hazard to health.

9 So a beer belly is much more dangerous than fat on your thighs or chest, and a waist bigger than 94 cm (about 37 inches) is a potential danger to your health, whatever your BMI. Above 102 cm (around 40 inches) and the risk that your weight will endanger your health increases dramatically[10]. Indeed, many experts believe that GPs should base their treatment for obesity and related-diseases on waist circumference rather than BMI[11]. But you should see your doctor if your BMI is 30 or over, if your waist circumference is more than 37 inches, or both.

10 Before you see your doctor, try to lose weight yourself first. Follow a calorie counted diet, cut back on the fat and eat plenty of fruit and vegetables, for example. And watch the alcohol. You could also try joining a club such as Weight Watchers, although it's probably best to steer clear of the latest celebrity endorsed fad diet. If watching what you eat still fails to get you back within the 'safe' zone, ask your doctor for advice[12].

11 Your doctor may take several measurements other than BMI and ask some questions. He or she will probably measure your blood pressure, for example. Nearly one in four adults in the UK has high blood pressure (hypertension)[13] that markedly increases their risk of suffering from a stroke or heart attack. And overweight men are between two and six times more likely to develop hypertension than the general population. Your doctor may also measure your waist because men with larger waists are carrying more visceral fat and are at an even higher risk of developing hypertension[14].

12 Taking drugs to lower raised blood pressure seems to reduce the risk of a stroke by more than 40%[15] and the risk of heart disease by about 14%. Unfortunately, high blood pressure rarely causes symptoms and most people are unaware that they have the disease. Doctors sometimes call hypertension the silent killer. And according to the British Heart Foundation, over a third of people with high blood pressure are not treated for hypertension[16]. So if your doctor doesn't measure your blood pressure, it's a good idea to ask.

13 Your doctor may also measure levels of glucose in your blood. This helps determine if you suffer from insulin resistance or type II diabetes (see Chapter 6). Losing weight can reduce your risk of suffering from diabetes. Your GP will probably also ask how much alcohol you drink. Drinking more than the recommended amount drives your blood pressure up[17], piles on the pounds and can lead to liver damage and other health problems.

14 You will probably also be asked if you smoke. Smoking dramatically increases your risk of suffering heart disease and makes other risk factors much more dangerous. Your doctor can prescribe several drugs that help determined people to quit smoking. For example, nicotine replacement therapy – patches and gums for example – roughly double your chance of quitting[18]. Another drug called bupropion helps some people quit.

Drugs that help you lose weight

15 Over recent years, doctors have been able to prescribe a growing number of drugs to help people who failed to lose weight on a calorie controlled diet.

16 One type of drug blocks one of the enzymes that digests fat so you absorb less fat from your diet. You then get rid of the excess when you defecate. You lose weight because fat is rich in calories and your body is digesting less of it. Another type of drug changes the levels of certain chemicals in the part of your brain that controls appetite. This means you feel full sooner and so you eat less.

In 1998, 17% of men – almost one in five – in England were obese and another 32% – around a third – were overweight, but not obese. So about half of men are either overweight or obese – that's three times more than in 1980, when just 6% of men were obese. If this rate continues, a quarter of us will be obese by 2010*.

* National Audit Commission Tackling Obesity in England 2001 p11-12.

17 Doctors should be able to prescribe several other drugs over the next few years. One of these, due to become available in 2006, helps rebalance your body's supply and demand for energy and helps regulate glucose and fat levels. Users lose weight and, in particular, the dangerous abdominal fat.

The Magic Mirror Technique

This is a very powerful way of setting personal change in motion that only takes a few minutes to do. Imagine that you are standing with a full length mirror behind you. Now imagine all those aspects of yourself that you no longer want, reflected in the mirror behind you. For example, you might imagine yourself as overweight (perhaps eating junk food); or as a smoker (perhaps with cigarettes in your mouth); or as somebody who is unfit, unhappy, or whatever. Spend a minute to allow yourself to notice all sorts of details about this image. Now imagine a full length mirror in front of you, and in this mirror see reflected the 'new you' that you want to become. Make this image as bright and realistic as possible. Imagine that you are smiling and happy, more confident, fitter, slimmer. You can imagine the clothes you are wearing, the way that you stand, the way you breathe and move. When this image is at its best, imagine that you step forward into it, and that you truly become the 'new you'. Notice how good you feel; be aware of how different you feel. Allow yourself to really enjoy this experience, to really live it. When you are ready, open your eyes again, and allow yourself to come back to the here-and-now. To really reinforce this work, repeat the whole process five more times, opening your eyes between each repetition.

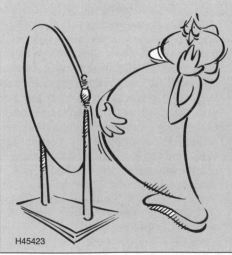

H45423

Cholesterol levels improve and the risk of developing the highly dangerous metabolic syndrome also declines, which should reduce the risk of suffering a heart attack or developing diabetes.

18 A couple of other points are worth mentioning. Firstly, all these drugs are used with a calorie controlled diet. And if you don't lose about 10% of your weight within a year, your doctor may stop treatment. So take your medicine and follow your diet plan.

19 Secondly, despite the temptations of e-mail spam, never buy any medicines – or indeed any herbal treatments that are supposed to lead to a dramatic weight loss – on line. Some may be counterfeit and there is a risk that you could put yourself at harm. These drugs are not suitable for everyone.

20 If drugs fail, you doctor may discuss surgery, especially if you are morbidly obese. Surgery is, however, a last resort and you should carefully weigh up the pros and cons with your doctor. Weight loss surgery takes one of two approaches. Firstly, surgeons can close off or remove part of your stomach. This means that your stomach can hold less food. Alternatively, surgeons can bypass the stomach or part of the intestines. So you absorb less food. Obviously, weight loss surgery is potentially dangerous. It really is the last resort when all else fails (see Chapter 2 for more about surgery).

References

1 Chambers R and Wakley G Obesity and Overweight Matters In Primary Care Radcliffe Medical Press 2002 Oxford p8.

2 Chambers R and Wakley G Obesity and Overweight Matters in Primary Care Radcliffe Medical Press 2002 Oxford p8.

3 Chambers R and Wakley G Obesity and Overweight Matters in Primary Care Radcliffe Medical Press 2002 Oxford Box 4.5.

4 http://www.bbc.co.uk/bigchallenge/challenges/3.shtml.

5 Chambers R and Wakley G Obesity and Overweight Matters in Primary Care Radcliffe Medical Press 2002 Oxford p4-5.

6 Chambers R and Wakley G Obesity and Overweight Matters in Primary Care Radcliffe Medical Press 2002 Oxford table 1.1.

7 http://nhlbisupport.com/bmi/bmicalc.htm

8 Chambers R and Wakley G Obesity and Overweight Matters in Primary Care Radcliffe Medical Press 2002 Oxford table 1.1.

9 Chambers R and Wakley G Obesity and Overweight Matters in Primary Care Radcliffe Medical Press 2002 Oxford p1.

10 Chambers R and Wakley G Obesity and Overweight Matters in Primary Care Radcliffe Medical Press 2002 Oxford table 1.2.

11 Chambers R and Wakley G Obesity and Overweight Matters in Primary Care Radcliffe Medical Press 2002 Oxford p1-2.

12 Wiseman G Nutrition & Health Taylor & Francis 2002 Table 10.

13 http://www.bhf.org.uk/hearthealth/index.asp?secondlevel=78&thirdlevel=169&artID=467.

14 Miller M and Vogel RA The Practice of Coronary Disease Prevention Williams & Wilkins 1996 p108.

15 Miller M and Vogel RA The Practice of Coronary Disease Prevention Williams & Wilkins 1996 p110.

16 http://www.bhf.org.uk/hearthealth/index.asp?secondlevel=78&thirdlevel=169&artID=467.

17 Miller M and Vogel RA The Practice of Coronary Disease Prevention Williams & Wilkins 1996 p108.

18 George TP and O'Malley SS Current pharmacological treatments for nicotine dependence Trends Pharmacol Sci 2004;25;43. figure based on cited Odds Ratios: 1.5–2.5.

Scottish men and those living in the North of England are especially likely to die from heart disease. About 50% more men die prematurely from heart disease in Scotland compared to the South West*.

* www.heartstats.org p13.

3 Metabolic syndrome

Bad luck comes in threes not pears

1 When it comes to waists, things going pear shaped are not nearly so bad as going apple shaped according the latest reports on the impact of obesity on health. If you look more like a Golden Delicious than a Bartlett you could be in trouble and are probably a man. Syndrome X sounds a bit spooky, sort of thing the X Files might suffer from but unlike the stuff agents Scully and Mulder investigated this threat is very real and far from being mere science fiction.

2 Better known as 'metabolic syndrome' it represents a greater threat to people of the developed world than any alien could begin to dream of. Obesity is now the greatest single danger to health in affluent societies like Britain, according to the World Health Organisation. Worse still they reckon that for the first time ever

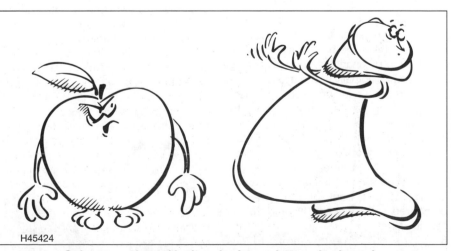

H45424

Going pear shaped isn't as bad as going apple shaped

today's children will have a lower life expectancy than their parents.

3 Metabolic syndrome is linked to obesity and is particularly nasty because it is almost silent. We were never aware of just how bad the situation really was until medical scientists recently revealed its true capacity to endanger life. It is a combination of three major risk factors.

4 Professor Tony Barnett from Birmingham's premier university describes metabolic syndrome as 'Obesity linked with two or more of the major cardiovascular risk factors' such as:
- *Hypertension (high blood pressure)*.
- *Dyslipidaemia (a dangerous change in the amount and type of fat in the blood)*.
- *Lowered ability to control blood sugar levels*.

5 It is estimated that in the USA the metabolic syndrome affects approximately 47 million people and that of these 20% will go on to develop type II diabetes.

6 Professor Barnett warns that if you're a woman with a bigger than 32 in waistline or a man with a bigger than 37 in measurement, you have an increased risk of diabetes and heart disease. At a London conference he told his audience of concerned health professionals that women a waist size of 35 in and men with 40 in versions face a four times greater risk of developing diabetes. An estimated 28 per cent of men and 20 per cent of women in the UK are now in the high risk category and it is on the increase.

Busts, buses and sabre tooth tigers

7 A woman's body is genetically designed to need fat that is slow-burning, particularly thigh and bottom fat, to sustain her through pregnancy and breastfeeding. Many women actually notice a loss of thigh fat during breastfeeding. Men don't need to store long term energy sources for obvious reasons. They only need ready supplies of quick-release fat to facilitate chasing sabre toothed tigers, or more likely these days the number 27 bus. So men tend to carry slightly less fat than women, around 20 per cent of body weight, compared with between 20 and 25 per cent in women.

8 Why should it be dangerous to look like a Granny Smith rather than be a granny? Apparently, unlike the stomach, fat cells on the thighs and hips tend to be quite inactive and don't produce so much toxic chemical and hormones that interfere with the body's systems. "Stomach fat cells produces chemicals, some of which seem to produce an imbalance of proteins and hormones that can damage the body's insulin system, putting you at risk of type II diabetes." said Prof Barnett. "On the plus side, stomach fat is busy and active so is actually easier to reduce than hip and thigh fat. In other words, your shape can change dramatically without too much effort".

9 Like in the States, a recent study of 38,000 adults in Britain found more and more of us turning into apples. The survey revealed that the most apple-shaped men in the country are to be found in north-west England (the average male waistband there is 37 in) but there are far more of them everywhere than before.

10 Although women have traditionally been pear-shaped, with most of their fat stored on their hips and thighs, the survey found a growing number of women are becoming apples. Women are now eating too much, exercising too little, and spilling out in the middle just like men.

11 It's not only your measurement in inches that's important but rather your waist-to-hip ratio calculated by dividing the waist by the hip measurement. According to dieticians, having a greater than 0.95 ratio if you are male or a 0.85 ratio if you're female makes you a less healthy shape. Men are often slim-waisted in youth but, like women, tend to lay down more fat in later life so watching your shape gets more important with birthdays.

Deaths from cardiovascular disease fell by 36% since the early 1990s. Mortality is extremely high in Central and Eastern Europe. But among economically developed countries only Ireland and Finland have higher rates of heart disease than the UK*.

* www.heartstats.org p13.

Keeping pear shaped

12 There is no shortage of advice on how to lose weight, diets range from eating only cabbage to drinking only fruit juice. Few succeed and can actually be dangerous. Most dieticians agree that a combination of increased activity along with reducing calorie intake over an long period is the only safe and effective way to lose weight, keep it off and return to pear shape. On the other hand eating apples and for that matter pears also makes sense as with all fruit and vegetables they will protect you from heart disease and some cancers. What is vital is to adopt a way of life which will enable you to keep the weight off rather than the short term quick fix solutions. Severe diets like Atkin's can produce dramatic results but as the body slips further and further into 'starvation mode' it will lay fat down much faster than normal once the diet is stopped and most people can only bear it for a limited period of time.

13 If you are very overweight you should talk to your doctor and get yourself on a controlled weight reduction programme.

14 Being a pear is much more fun, lasts longer and doesn't leave a nasty taste in your mouth like a crab apple!

Benefits in a 10 kg/22lb excess weight loss in the population	
Death rates	20-25% fall in total premature deaths
	30-40% fall in diabetes related deaths
	40-50% fall in obesity related cancer deaths
Blood Pressure	Fall of about 10 units of blood pressure
Angina (chest pain from the heart)	Reduced symptoms by 91%
	33% increase in exercise tolerance
Lipids (fats in the blood)	Fall of 10% total cholesterol (bad fat)
	Fall of 15% LDL cholesterol (bad fat)
	Fall of 30% triglycerides (bad fat)
	Increase of 8% HDL cholesterol (good fat)
Diabetes	Reduces risk of developing diabetes by over 50%

4 Eat more, weigh less – is the Low Carb choice for you?

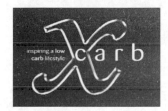

1 There is seemingly a simple solution that has been around for a very long time, yet only of late, has gripped the attention of the western world. In the last couple of years low carbohydrate, high-protein eating plans, originally created back in 1863, are now embraced by a previously sceptical public. Ironically, it was a male behind the diet revolution, with William Banting writing one of the most famous books on obesity to this day. He ultimately changed the thinking on diets and this is now paving the way for men watching their weight.

The Thinking Behind Low-Carb

2 There are so many different diets being concocted and messages being disseminated every day of our lives. The task of knowing which diet option is the right one can be baffling. Even low-carb dieting has its many options and requires varying amounts of carbs, protein and fat.

So how do carbs work?

3 Whichever low carb eating plan is the right one for you, the common theme is that if you eat high amounts of carbohydrate, this in turn causes an overproduction of insulin which leads to overeating, obesity and insulin resistance. A reduction in carbs is necessary for most in today's society due to the amount of processed foods that we are all eating; however the right carbs are still important as they:

- Are the main source of fuel for the body.
- Are quickly and easily used by the body for energy.
- Can be stored in the muscles for exercise.
- Provide lots of vitamins, minerals and fibre.
- Help your body function properly without fatigue.

4 The trick is to choose the right kinds of carbs (see complex and simple) and, of course, eat a reasonable amount of them as too many (as with too much of anything) can be stored as fat.

Simple carbs

5 Chocolate and fizzy drinks are quickly digested and can be used immediately for energy. However, they spike blood glucose levels, which then lead to a crash when blood sugar drops. Simple carbs (such as raisins) can be a good option before going to the gym, but consumed merely as a snack can lead to a feeling of lethargy.

Complex carbs

6 Take longer to digest and come from whole grain products, pulses, and fruits. They are slowly released into the body, unlike simple carbs, so there is no immediate sugar rush or crash. Complex carbs are almost always the best choice, even for low carbers because they are naturally low in fat, high in fibre and provide vitamins and minerals.

> Men with manual jobs are 58% more likely to die prematurely from heart disease than their white collar counterparts*.
>
> * www.heartstats.org p13.

So what defines 'Low-Carb'?

7 There are many different low carb diets in the public domain being followed by celebrity after celebrity; however it is vital each individual diet is understood prior to merely following a trend as they all recommend a different level of carb intake. The most popular choices at the moment seem to be the Zone, the South Beach and the more extreme Atkins. The following points should give an indication into the difference of suggested requirements:

- The National Academy of Sciences recommends no less than 120 grams of carbs per day.
- The recommended daily allowance (RDA) is 300 grams of carbs per 2000 calories.
- Diets such as the Atkins initially recommends 20 grams per day.
- The Zone advises keeping carbs at 40% of total calories.

8 While we don't know which diet is the right one for any given individual, recent studies at the University of Connecticut, found that low carbohydrate diets, like the South Beach Diet, may actually be the best option for men who want to stay in shape.

9 The research showed that over 70 percent of men lost more weight and fat on a low carbohydrate diet, despite eating more calories. It also found that fat loss in men was three-times greater in the trunk area, when they were on a low-carbohydrate regime compared to a low-fat diet.

Mythunderstood – cutting through the mystique of Low Carb

10 Low carb eating is not rocket science and can be beneficial when followed correctly. As with anything, problems could arise if a low carber is misinformed, or when simple common sense is discarded.

11 Hopefully, the following will help cut through some of the myths and provide the know-how to make low carb the right choice:

Myth: Low carb foods are the solution to obesity

Fact: Lowering carbs can play a part in an overall effort to lose weight, however limiting them alone will not undo a collection of other dietary downfalls, or make up for a lack of physical activity. Successful weight loss and weight maintenance depends on the right balance of diet and physical activity.

Myth: Low-carb means low calorie or high fat

Fact: Not in most cases, however there is an increasingly wide choice of low carb foods focusing on keeping calorific and fat content to a minimum. These offer convenience and in some notable cases, taste; covering breakfast, lunch, dinner and snacking on the go, making a low carb lifestyle easy to follow.

Myth: Low carb (or any diet) equals no taste

Fact: Diet products are more often than not somewhat less than satisfying. However, the commitment to making good-tasting, low carb foods is clearly evident in today's marketplace with the emergence of product ranges resulting in some undeniably tasty products.

Myth: You can't eat vegetables

Fact: Even on the most restrictive of the major low-carb diets, they not only permit vegetables, but encourage their consumption. Regardless of which low-carb diet you choose, the trick is choosing the right veggies, such as broccoli, cauliflower, tomatoes and many more.

Myth: It's worked for everybody I know so it should work for me as well

Fact: Everyone is different and it is important to understand all the pros and cons. From that, an informed decision can be made whether to restrict carbs based on personal goals and health status.

No one method will suit everyone. In reality, you may find that combining several aspects of these different approaches works for you. If you can enjoy a new way of cooking and eating, are not going hungry and are still losing one pound per week then that is the right way for you.

Step one

Cut out the junk	**Try**
Chocolate bars, crisps, 'junk' food, chips	Fizzy mineral water
Cola and other soft drinks	Squares of 70% cocoa chocolate
Reduce alcohol intake	Mints (in moderation)
	Fresh fruit – apples, oranges, pears, grapes, tangerines, pineapple, mango. Some are higher in carbohydrates than others (eg, mango, grapes)
	Fresh nuts

Step two

Reduce fat intake	**Try**
Ready meals	Semi-skimmed milk, and reduced or low fat dairy products
Take-away meals	Look at the label on packet foods – always aim for less than 5% fat content. Sometimes more expensive, usually better value (fat is used as cheap 'padding' for foods)
Meals out	Cook 'in' more often – eg, learn to cook Chinese 'stir fries', make your own pizzas, or do pan-fried fish (buy a good, heavy, non-stick frying pan) – buy some new cookery books
Dairy products	
Processed meat products	
Cakes, biscuits and pastries (high 'hidden' fat content)	

Step three

Reduce high 'GI' carbs	**Try**
White bread	Heavier breads – eg, whole meal, wheaten or rye (buy a bread maker?!)
Baked or mashed potatoes	Pasta (try low carb varieties)
Some breakfast cereals (especially with added sugar)	Any fresh fruit or vegetables (but some are higher in carbs, eg, mango, grapes)
White rice	Basmati rice
Biscuits and cakes	Porridge
High sugar products	Cauliflower, peas, peanuts, broccoli. These will complement any high protein foods – eggs, yoghurt (and cheese), chicken, fish, red meat (in moderation). It is always best to trim excess fat from meat, or to drain fat when cooked

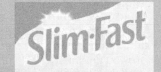

There's a simple, foolproof way to lose weight that takes the thinking out of losing – it's been used by millions of people over the past 25 years, has the support of the US and European scientific community, has helped people keep weight off for as long as 10 years and can show that when used properly it stopped a whole community in Wisconsin from gaining weight like the rest of America.

What is this simple miracle then?

It's meal replacements.

Now, how dull does that sound? But never mind the dull, watch the waistband!

Just like it said in the old ads (when you and me were young and spent a small amount of time wondering who was this Barry Bethel nagging us on TV who used to be so fat and was now so slim) "a shake for breakfast, a shake for lunch and a sensible dinner in the evening".

Ever since Barry's immortal words on TV more than 15 years ago, slimming diets have come and gone but meal replacements are still there – reliable, effective and (while they may not be a whole lot of fun) so simple that you can't lose – or perhaps better put – all you can do is lose!

So what are they?

They're usually shakes or bars. Basically, without going into too much detail, they've got the nutrition of something like a 600 calorie meal packed into around 200 calories – so you get the protein, the vitamins and minerals and stuff – and all you dump is the calories. You have one instead of breakfast, another instead of lunch, and a good, low fat, balanced meal in the evening.

It means you don't have to count or think about breakfast and lunch, and if you're well set up and organised you can even get someone else to cook the sensible dinner for you!.

If you're a particularly big fellow you'll need more than just two meal replacements to keep going – so treat yourself to a third during the day, or add fruit and veg as snacks between meals.

The whole point of the meal replacement diet is that it's really simple:

• *You don't have to think about what to eat for breakfast and lunch.*
• *You can take meal replacements around with you – to work or for a day out.*

It's a real no-brainer of a way to manage your weight.

And after you've lost the weight – keep it off like the folk in Wisconsin by replacing that lunchtime sandwich and crisps with a good old meal replacement shake.

For more information about the Slim Fast Plan go to www.slimfast.co.uk. For specific enquiries ring 0845 6001311 or e-mail: slimfast@unileverconsumerlink.co.uk

5 The importance of water in our diet

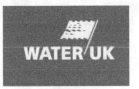

• Water is one of the six basic nutrients. Since the body requires it constantly and all the important chemical reactions – such as the production of energy – take place in water, it is widely seen as the most important.
• Water is the main constituent of the body and forms 50-60% of body weight. The exact amount varies with age and sex and also depends on body fat content.
• Water contains no fats, no proteins, no carbohydrates and therefore no calories.
• Water is the perfect complement for a nutritionally balanced meal.
• Fluid loss corresponding to 2.5% of body weight has been shown to reduce physical performance capacity by 45%.

• Even in the absence of any visible perspiration, approximately half of water loss occurs through the operation of our lungs and skin.
• In hot climates and during heavy exercise, sweating rates can be as high as 2500 ml/hr. Water loss of 500ml/hour is not unusual.
• If you exercise to burn off fat and keep trim, there is little point working off the calories just to replace them with a high sugar sports drink. When you are exercising for durations of an hour or less – and this applies to elite athletes just as much as fitness fans – cool, fresh water is the only drink you need. A suitably balanced diet will take care of the rest.
• Remember also that sugar slows down the rate at which water can be absorbed from the stomach.
• When we stand on the scales after moderate exercise and note that we have achieved a weight loss, it is normally dehydration rather than loss of fat – your body weight will return as you re-hydrate your body.
• When the body is not adequately hydrated, it responds by conserving its stocks, shifting water to where it is most needed and causing thirst.

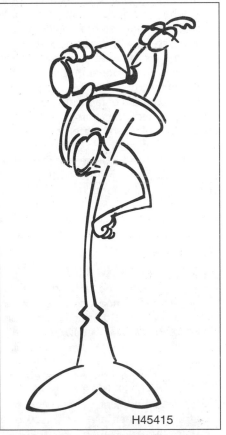

H45415

When exercising, remember to keep hydrated

Water facts versus water myths

- Ten litres of tap water costs around one penny – that can be as much as 1000 times cheaper than bottled water.
- Tap water in the UK is amongst the highest quality in the world.
- We each use around 150 litres of water each day, but national surveys show us that we drink as little as one litre – around half the recommended daily amount.
- There are no health advantages to drinking expensive bottled water instead of water from your tap.
- Tap water tastes best when it is served fresh and served cool.
- It is recommended that adults should drink around two litres of water daily, and consider more when they perform exercise and/or the weather is hot.

Ten Tips for drinking more water

1 All relevant medical practice and care guidance must be observed before considering these suggestions.
- In a sedentary day, try to drink around 2 litres of water.
- Start by drinking a glass of fresh water when you get up in the morning.
- If you are not used to drinking water regularly, try initially replacing just one of your other drinks a day with fresh water, increasing your consumption as the weeks go by.
- Ask for a glass of tap water to go with your coffee and tea in cafes.
- Drink a glass of water before and during each meal.
- Hot water with a piece of fruit in – like lemon, lime, orange, etc – often helps those who want a hot drink.
- Carry a bottle filled with chilled tap water with you whenever you leave the house.

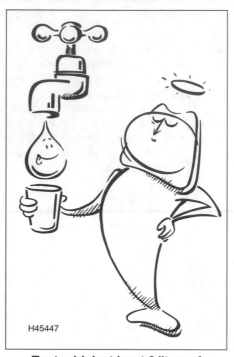

Try to drink at least 2 litres of water a day

- During exercise, drink at 10 to 15 minutes intervals or think of it as a full glass every 30 minutes – drink slowly and drink early, it's physically easier to do this when you are still feeling fresh.
- Keep a check on your urine. As a general guide to hydration, it should be plentiful, pale in colour and odourless.
- Ask for a jug of iced tap water with your meal when in restaurants and with your alcohol when in bars – good establishments will be happy to provide this.

The FA's key hydration tips for athletes

- If you finish a training session and you are thirsty, then you have not taken enough fluid on board during the session. Whenever you become thirsty, start to drink immediately. Preferably, drink before you are thirsty.
- Rehydration is a major part of the recovery process after exercise, but little attention has been paid by players and coaches to the need to adequately rehydrate in order to perform optimally during subsequent exercise bouts.
- It is well established that exercise performance is seriously impaired in a dehydrated state (a 2% decrease in body weight can lead to a greater than 30% fall in performance) and that both high-intensity and endurance activities are affected. There is also an increased risk of heat illness in individuals who begin exercise in a dehydrated state.
- Rehydration requires replacement of body water loss, but ingestion of plain water is not an effective way to achieve a positive state of hydration. Drinks should contain moderately high levels of sodium and possibly some potassium.
- To surmount ongoing urine losses, the volume consumed should be greater than the volume of sweat lost. Palatability of beverages is an important factor in stimulating drinking.

6 Policemen and nutrition

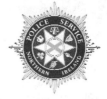

POLICE SERVICE of NORTHERN IRELAND

Case history

1 The criteria for recruits into the RIC (Royal Irish Constabulary) in 1911 read 'persons must be at least five foot nine inches in height, strong and active, a single man between the ages of nineteen and twenty seven … of good physique to warrant their admission'. They were also on the look out for men with a chest measurement of at least 37 ins. Since then, there have been many changes in policing, women are now allowed onto

Water: more than just a prefix

Men are keen on sheds; garden sheds, potting sheds, railway sheds and especially watersheds, as life events are important rites to passage.

Without water it is calculated the average UK male would lose around 450 words from his everyday vocabulary. Feet slipping off bicycle pedals would then become "it certainly made my eyes something". Electricians would get sick notes from their doctor saying, "Mr Smith has something on the knee". It is also a handy fluid substitute for tea, coffee or real ale.

Most men should drink far more unadulterated water, not least as it helps the body flush out toxins generally consumed in exactly the opposite manner. Which is strange as men are composed of around 98% water rather than 'Hogshead Winter Warmer'. Perhaps on occasion us Y chromosome owners need a good tap on the head.

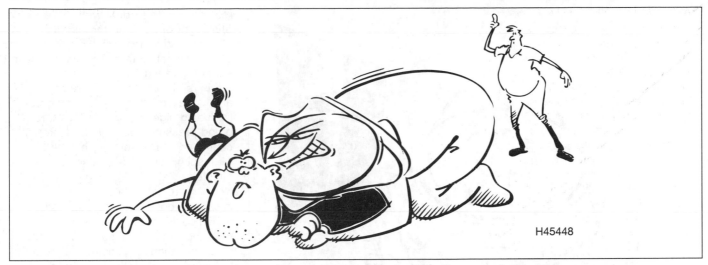

H45448

A hundred years ago the policeman on the beat had a more physical job

the force, older recruits are accepted and generally it's overall body composition that the medical officers are interested in.

2 In the early twentieth century policing was a physically demanding job. It used to be that policemen would not have to worry about their weight as they were either walking for miles and miles on the beat in all sorts of weather or cycling around the community, keeping a check on their local area. Physical confrontation happened regularly and the peeler had to be able to defend himself. It's all different now – the main method of transport is 4 wheels instead of 2 and much of the job is deskbound with the increase in paperwork. Just as the UK diet has changed in that time from one of locally produced, quality food, to a nation of fast food, so too has what is on offer in the police canteens. The food that sells is the cheap, nutritionally devoid junk food like chips, burgers, sausage rolls and fizzy drinks. Most of the canteens do offer a good healthy option, such as baked potatoes, salads, fish, etc, it's just that police officers do not tend to select the healthy choice.

3 Modern recruits are still expected to pass a demanding fitness test and the first few weeks in the training college are both physically and mentally challenging. However once policemen have passed this initiation, there is no incentive for them to be lean, mean machines. Most cops end up in a station where the temptation is a big fry-up for breakfast, chips for lunch and chocolate and

crisps with endless mugs of coffee for snacks.

4 Police are notorious for their eating habits – it used to be that police who worked overtime would be given a meal ticket for the police canteen – these became known as 'white fivers' and rumour had it that they were even accepted at the local Chinese takeaway!

5 Approximately 80-90% of police work is now sedentary[1]. It is assumed that police officers should be well above average in all physical attributes – bigger, faster, stronger... but, in reality he is just an average guy, with the same weighty concerns as any member of the public.

Fat boy slim?

6 So how would you fare as a police recruit nowadays?[2] Instead of taking your chest measurements, you are more likely to have your body fat percentage surveyed and your BMI and hip:waist ratio calculated (see Chapter 5).

7 The main problem with using the BMI is that it doesn't take into account whether you are big because you are fat, or big because you are muscular. So a very fit tactical support officer might have a BMI of 30 or more, but be built like a brickhouse, whereas his unfit and overweight colleague working in at a desk job might have the same BMI, but be built more like a blancmange.

8 That's why other measurements are often used alongside the BMI. Another measurement you can easily assess yourself on is your waist circumference.

Men should measure up less than 102cms round the middle.

9 It has been found that policemen over 36 years of age are significantly fatter than their younger counterparts. There could be a number of reasons for this – not least a lack of exercise and promotion to a more sedentary job than men in their younger years[3].

Diet squad

10 We all know that the recipe for weight management is healthy eating combined with regular exercise. Sounds easy – but whether you are a policeman on the beat or spend most of your working day at a desk, whether it is the aroma of a cooked breakfast or the sweet treats that appeal, temptation will be all around to lead you off the straight and narrow.

11 A few simple diet laws can help you crack the bad habits and downsize the belly. The key to a successful weight loss programme is something that fits the following criteria:

- *Easy to stick to.*
- *Keeps hunger at bay.*
- *Get results – the weight will come off and stay off.*
- *Nutritious and delicious foods.*
- *Makes you feel good.*

Policing your metabolism

12 Weight management is just a matter of choosing the right foods. It is not uncommon to hear an officer order a fry up with the works – double sausage, bacon, eggs (fried of course), soda bread and all the condiments and then ask for a

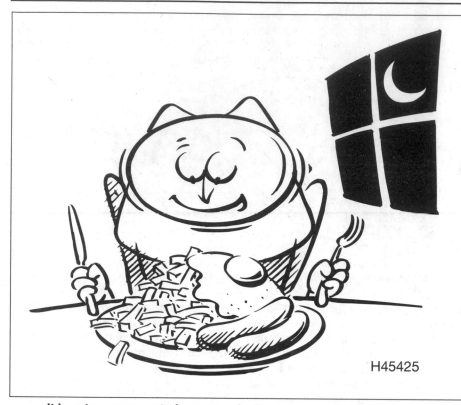

It is not uncommon to hear an order for a fry up with the works . . .

H45425

diet coke with it. It is going to take a little bit more than this to fight the fat.

13 Your goal for weight loss should be about 1-2lbs a week. If you lose weight faster than this, it is just water loss, which will come back just as quickly as it went.

14 In theory, the calories you take in through your diet, less the calories you burn off through exercise ends up as excess flab. But this doesn't take into account how the body deals with fuel – in other words, your metabolic rate. We all use energy at different rates – some people can eat whatever they want and never put on weight, while others just need to look at food to pile on the pounds. So the key to effective weight loss is boosting your metabolism – which is why exercise is so important. But, you can also regulate your metabolic rate by adopting the correct diet enforcement strategy.

15 If you have ever been on a low calorie diet, you will know that your body soon compensates for the food shortage by slowing down your metabolic rate, so although the diet may work for the first short while, as soon as you go back to your regular eating habits, the weight returns – with a vengeance! So each time you diet it gets harder and harder to shift

the weight and instead of getting thinner, you end up worse off than when you started.

Fight the insulin resistance

16 You can't have failed to notice the shift away from low fat to high protein/low carb diets for weight loss recently. The problem is neither of these diets is sustainable in the long term. The human body is designed to use carbohydrate as its primary fuel source. So if you deprive yourself of carbohydrate, you will soon deprive yourself of energy too.

17 The key to controlling weight, stopping cravings and feeling good is insulin. Insulin is a hormone produced by your pancreas that polices the levels of sugar in the bloodstream. The more sugar you eat the more insulin your pancreas produces and the more fat you store. Insulin also stops fat breakdown, so once these stores are laid down it is hard to get rid of them if your insulin levels are to remain high.

18 If you are constantly snacking on sugary foods, drinking tea or coffee and eating fast foods or ready meals, your pancreas is under stress to continually

release insulin to deal with this steady onslaught of sugar in the bloodstream. The longer this goes on, the slower your body's response rate. Eventually insulin stops regulating your blood sugar levels – this is known as insulin resistance – and one of the major symptoms (including high triglyceride levels, raised blood pressure and high cholesterol) is central adiposity – or belly blubber.

19 Insulin levels are also adversely affected by stress. Policing (especially in Northern Ireland over the last 30+ years) is seen as one of the most stressful jobs a man could choose, so the chances are more policemen will suffer from insulin resistance than the estimated 40% of the UK adult population affected. This condition is attributed solely to crimes in diet and physical activity habits[4]. Managing blood sugar levels will control insulin response, boost your metabolism and fight the flab. There are just a few simple diet laws you need to follow:

The law abiders

- *Eat small, regular balanced meals.*
- *Run your body on the right fuel.*
- *Cut the stimulants.*
- *Have some protein with each meal.*
- *Eat fat to beat fat.*
- *Rehydrate the body with 2 litres of water a day.*

Diet criminals

- *Fast food.*
- *Eating on the run.*
- *Convenience foods.*
- *Sugary or fatty snacks.*
- *Lack of fresh fruit and vegetables.*
- *Dehydration.*
- *Skipping meals.*
- *Caffeine.*

Eat small regular meals

20 To lose weight and keep it off, it is crucial that you are eating at regular intervals. So graze, don't gorge! Grazing on the right sort of foods keeps hunger at bay and blood sugar levels regulated. If you go too long without eating, the body thinks it is in a state of starvation, so your metabolic rate will slow down to compensate. So as a general rule, you should be eating about every three to four hours, even if you are on nights and the canteen is shut. But... this does not mean your hand should be in the biscuit tin every few hours. Check out the ideas below for an idea of nutritious and delicious snacks:

- Oatcakes with houmous (a Middle Eastern dip made from chickpeas, sesame seeds, olive oil and garlic) or low fat cheese.
- A handful of unsalted and unroasted nuts (like hazelnuts, brazils, walnuts, pecans or almonds) with a piece of fruit.
- A small pot of natural yoghurt – flavoured yoghurts and low fat yoghurts are often loaded with sugar, so steer clear of them.
- A fruit smoothie: really easy to make, even in the station kitchen. All you need is some natural yoghurt, milk and some soft fruit like a banana, peach, kiwi, mango – or a combination of any fruits you fancy – if you have a freezer in your station, you could use frozen berries. Just whiz the lot up in a blender. Alternatively you could make this up at home and bring it into work in a flask.
- Wholegrain bread with no-added-sugar peanut butter (some companies make great nut butters – almond, cashew, peanut... try them – you might even find you like them.)

The right fuel: boy racers & Sunday drivers

21 Carbohydrate is the body's primary fuel source. Sources of carbohydrate include bread, pasta, potatoes and rice. It's just a case of taking in the right sort of carbohydrate through your diet for optimum efficiency and peak performance.

22 Carbohydrate is broken down into sugar in the bloodstream. The rate at which it is released, determines whether is will end up as a wedge of fat around your middle, or help to keep your energy levels sustained and even throughout the day. Generally speaking, anything that is white, refined, processed, sweet or sugary is a fast release carbohydrate. Anything that is whole, unprocessed, fibre-rich and unrefined is a slow release carbohydrate.

23 Think about your bloodstream as a motorway. Different foods will be travelling at different speeds down this road. So the fast release carbs are like boy racers – they are travelling far too fast through your bloodstream, so they upset the balance and you end up

gaining points (or pounds). On the other hand, the law abiders are the slow release foods. They will get to their destination efficiently and without causing havoc en route.

24 Sugars, white, refined and processed foods are like feeding your body with rocket fuel – they will give you a quick fix of energy, by initiating a spike in blood sugar levels, but will leave you feeling tired, fed up and overweight. The sugar rush initiates that release of insulin, which tells the body to store the sugar (energy) that you are not using as fat (energy stores).

25 On the other hand, unrefined, unprocessed and whole foods (whole foods are not just about brown rice and lentils – anything that has not been refined or processed is a whole food – even fruits and vegetables) are a more sustained energy source for your body. They will help to keep blood sugar levels stable, satisfy your hunger and stop the pounds piling on.

26 So the rules are simple – fast release carbohydrates result in a peak in insulin levels, which pile on the pounds, while slow release carbs are the sustained fuel your body prefers. So steer clear of the white rice, white pasta, sweets and chocolate and make the switch to wholegrain bread, brown rice, oats, etc.

27 The chart below gives you some ideas about the choices you could easily make at home or in the station's canteen.

Refined	Unrefined
Corn flakes	Muesli or porridge
White toast	Wholegrain or wheaten bread
Chocolate bar	Nut & seed bar or a piece of fruit with a handful of nuts or seeds
French bread	Wheaten bread
White pasta	Wholewheat pasta
Breadsticks	Oatcakes
White rice	Brown basmati rice

28 The key is to choose good sources of carbohydrate that contain fibre – the roughage will not only help to keep you regular in the digestive front, but also keep hunger at bay and blood sugar levels well balanced.

Cut the stimulants

29 Stimulants come in many guises – tea, coffee, colas, chocolate and some fizzy drinks are good sources. Just the thing to keep you awake when you are in the middle of a night shift or bogged down with boring paperwork. The

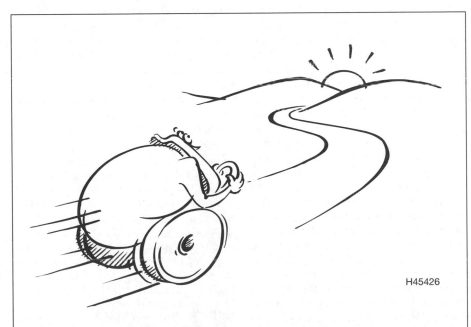

Think of the bloodstream as a motorway – slow-release carbs get to their destination efficiently and without causing havoc en route

problem is that stimulants also elicit an insulin response. They spark the adrenals into a state of fight-or-flight, to release adrenalin, which results in raised blood sugar levels, in turn triggering an insulin response.

30 With or without the sweet treat, caffeinated drinks cause a massive blood sugar fluctuation, which will upset insulin levels and make the battle of the bulge even harder to fight. So kick the habit and adopt healthier options. Try switching to decaf instead – or even better, give the herbal teas a go instead.

Have some protein with each meal

31 Having a little protein with each meal will help control the insulin release from the meal and so help you bust that gut. However some high protein foods are also high in saturated fat, so it is important you to make the right choice.

32 Good sources of protein include:
- Fish.
- Chicken.
- Lean red meat (1-2 times a week).
- Eggs.
- Nuts & seeds or nut butter.
- Low fat and low sugar dairy produce, eg, natural yoghurt, cottage cheese, semi skimmed milk.
- Beans and lentils.

33 As a general rule, a portion size of protein is about the size of a salmon steak or chicken breast. Try adding a handful of nuts (like almonds, brazils, hazelnuts) or seeds (like sunflower, pumpkin or sesame) to your breakfast cereal and always make sure lunch and dinner include something from the above list.

Eat fat to beat fat

34 Believe it or not, eating fat can actually help you lose weight. It's just a matter of choosing the right sort of fat. The essential fats for health are the omega 3 and omega 6 fats, found in oily fish, seeds (like sunflower, pumpkin and sesame seeds) and unroasted and unsalted nuts (brazils, almonds, hazelnuts, walnuts, etc). It seems that these fats can improve insulin resistance in the body and aid weight loss in overweight or obese individuals.

35 Men should be including oily fish (sardines, salmon, trout, herring or mackerel) in their diets four times a week and having a handful of nuts or seeds every day to comply with current recommendations (for women it's twice a week).

36 Tinned fish makes a handy snack to take into the station, especially for those officers who are working shifts and have limited access to the canteen – sardines on toasted wholegrain bread makes a perfect tasty and healthy snack. If you are choosing tinned fish, those tinned in olive oil, spring water or tomato sauce are best from a health point of view.

37 Sunflower, pumpkin and sesame seeds are the best dietary source of omega 6 fats – these can be mixed together and stored in a jar and added to porridge, yoghurts, salads or stir fries – or simply used as a handy snack – ideal for keeping in the glove box of the police vehicle if you are out and about.

38 If you have a look at some of what's on offer in the hot-food counter of the station canteen, a lot of this is the sort of fat you want to keep to a minimum. The menu is usually loaded with saturated and trans fats.

39 We all know about saturated fats – the diet police have told us often enough over the years how detrimental they are to our health. But you may not have heard of trans fats. Trans (or hydrogenated) fats are the terrorists of the diet world. They have been linked to an increase in obesity and heart disease. Recently the US government have forced food manufacturers to state the amount of trans fats on their products.

40 Trans fats are found in all processed foods where polyunsaturated fat has been subject to high temperatures. So anything that has been fried in sunflower or vegetable oil, which we are used to thinking of as the 'healthy' alternative, is really a health time bomb. Crisps, chips, chocolate bars, biscuits, processed foods, breads – these are all loaded with trans fats.

41 Trans fats are also found in a lot of margarines and low fat spreads. So opt for the healthier alternative and use a little butter (organic if possible) instead. Even though it is a saturated fat, it is a healthier alternative than the treacherous trans fats.

Rehydrate the body with 2 litres of water a day

42 Make sure you are not mistaking hunger pangs for thirst! We need to be taking about 2 litres of water on board every day for optimal health. Tea and coffee not only upset the insulin balance, but they also act as diuretics and so cause dehydration. So instead of always reaching for a cuppa, make sure you have a bottle of water either within reaching distance of your desk, or with you in the patrol vehicle to keep your levels topped up.

Booze watch

43 Policemen are social animals. For many officers, grabbing a coffee and a sandwich with colleagues or community workers, working undercover in pubs and clubs or dining at social functions are all part of the daily grind.

44 Then when they switch off after a hard day's work, there's nothing more they enjoy than a wind-down over an alcoholic beverage in the mess.

45 If you are expected to attend social functions at work, the message is to balance that out with regular exercise and healthy eating at other times. If you are lucky enough to be able to choose from the menu, opt for something like the soup or a salad for starters, followed by a main course of fish, chicken or even a lean steak – but just switch the chips for a salad for vegetable medley and then finish with a dessert of fruit salad. Of course alcohol just adds weight to the problem, or beer to the belly. So it is important to take it easy on the booze too.

Solving the crime

46 So the evidence suggests that the key to winning the war of terror on fat is to boost your metabolic rate through diet and regular exercise.

47 Remember, it's not just how much food you shove in your gob – it's also the sort of food you scoff that will help win the war on the fat.

48 By adopting a healthy approach to weight management, you can enjoy good food, control your appetite and beat the battle of the bulge – without much effort at all.

49 More fibre, slow release carbs, the right sort of fats and cutting the stimulants will keep energy levels more consistent, hunger at bay and help the body burn flab. The key to successful weight loss is a diet that you can stick to, one that is easy to do even when are cooking in the station's kitchen or choosing from the not-so-healthy canteen menu.

The chief inspectors

50 Here is your checklist for effective weight management.

- Exercise at least 5 times a week for 30 minutes.
- Graze, don't gorge – but choose your snacks wisely.
- Always eat breakfast (just stay away from the mega fry-ups and opt for a healthy cereal like muesli or porridge instead – or even choose some scrambled egg with wholegrain bread).
- Have some protein with each meal.
- Cut the stimulants.
- Drink at least one and a half litres of water every day.
- Stay away from the low fat foods – they are all too often loaded with sugar and additives.
- Make sure you are making the right choice of fats – eat oily fish 4 times a week & have a handful of seeds or nuts every day.

51 Keep a log of what you eat and when – use the food diary provided to help you – then become a diet detective and check each of the above off your daily list.

Did you know?[5]

- The biggest reason for police recruits being turned away from the RIC in the early 1900s was because of the state of their badly decayed teeth!
- 90% of new recruits into the RIC in 1911 stated their previous occupation as farmers or labourers. Most of these men were the second sons of local farmers who had lost out on inheriting the farm to their older brothers.
- UK men are fatter than UK women. 37% of men, compared with 24% women are overweight, but twice as many women as men are dieting (1 in 6 women at any one time)
- Obesity and a general lack of physical fitness are catching up with tobacco as the main causes of death in the USA.
- The only difference between brown bread and white bread is the colour? If a label reads *brown* bread, it has just had food colouring added to make it look more wholesome, so it is no more nutritionally beneficial than white

bread. Wholegrain or wholemeal bread on the other hand are made with the whole grain and so contain lots of fibre to keep you regular and satisfy your appetite.

Health statistics

- Just one in five people in Northern Ireland eat the recommended five or more portions of fruit and vegetables a day, but 44% of people surveyed eat biscuits very day!
- The main reason why people find it difficult to change their eating habits is lack of willpower (25%).
- Men in Northern Ireland were found to eat more chips, fried food, savoury snacks, such as crisps, and sugary fizzy drinks more often than women.
- Men aged 18-29 years are less aware of healthy eating messages and eat fewer of the foods recommended for health.
- A staggering 94% of people in the UK have doubts about the government's advice on food and obesity[6].
- Research shows that Brits pile on the pounds when they go on a diet instead of losing weight. 20% of people surveyed said that they ended up a stone heavier than when the diet started[7]!
- Over a quarter of the UK population are currently on a diet and approximately one in five adults in the UK are heavy enough to be putting their health at risk[8].
- Obesity has tripled in men since 1980.
- Brits are the biggest consumers of chocolate in Europe – we chomp our way through a mountain of 10 kgs per person per year! Britain is followed by Germany, Ireland and the Netherlands, while Spaniards nibble on just 1.7 kg per year[9].
- In the UK we also love our fizzy drinks – consuming more than 5560 million litres a year[10]. In May 2002, a survey for Highland Spring reported that a fifth of 7-10 year olds drink nearly 10 cans of fizzy a week (nearly 70 spoonfuls of sugar). An average can of fizzy has 7-8 spoonfuls of sugar…

Food Myths

Eating fat makes you fat

Eating plenty of the omega 3 and omega 6 essential fats can help your body burn fat.

Low fat foods can help you lose weight

The diet food industry has expanded hugely in the last 20 years or so – but so have our waistlines! This is because although these foods may be low in fat, many of them compensate by adding sugar, to appeal to our tastebuds. Sugar is THE biggest obstacle in the battle of the bulge.

Calorie counting is the best way to lose weight

Not only is calorie counting boring, but it doesn't work – it's hard to stick to and once you get back to eating normally you will pile the pounds back on, because your metabolism will have slowed down to compensate.

All calories are equal

Stop calorie counting – a calorie from a fat has a different physiological effect than a calorie from a protein that has a different physiological effect than a calorie from a carbohydrate. And then it depends whether it is an essential fat or a saturated fat, a simple carb or a complex carb… Not all calories will pile on the pounds.

Low calorie diets are the best way to lose weight

How many times have you heard the only way to lose weight is to eat less? In theory, the less you eat the better – but these low calorie diets are a disaster for weight management in the long haul. All they do is slow down your metabolism so as soon as you get back to your normal calorie intake, the pounds pile back on again – with a vengeance – making it harder and harder to lose the weight.

References

1 Bonneau J, Brown, J. Physical ability, fitness and police work. Journal of Clinical Forensic Medicine 1995; 2: 157-164.

2 Spitler DL et al. Body composition and physiological characteristics of law enforcement officers. British Journal of Sports Medicine 1987 Dec; 21 (4): 154-157.

3 Franke, WD & Anderson, DF (1994). Relationship between physical activity & risk factors for cardiovascular disease among law enforcement officers. Journal of occupational Medicine 36 (10); 1127-1132.

[4] Erica Weir & Lorraine Lipscombe Metabolic syndrome: Waist not, want not. CMAJ April 27,2004; 170 (9).

[5] First four from Eating for Health? A survey of attitudes, awareness and eating habits among adults in Northern Ireland. Health Promotion Agency for Northern Ireland.

[6] www.cambridge20.co.uk.

[7] www.bdaweightwise.com – British Dietetic Association.

[8] www.bdaweightwise.com – British Dietetic Association.

[9] www.foodnavigator.com

[10] bbc.co.uk/health

7   Men at work

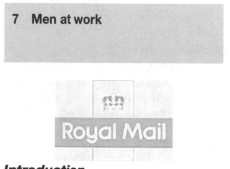

Introduction

1   Why did bus conductors have less heart problems than the driver of the bus? This difference was thought to be due to their different levels of physical activity. Physical activity is an important influence on the maintenance of body weight and the risks of diseases associated with obesity.

2   Working men have become heavier over the years reflecting changes in the general population. This is partly due to reducing physical activity at work and an ageing workforce. About 5% of men aged 16-24 years are obese but by age 55-64 years the rate has increased nearly five fold to 23%.

3   Work has got less physical as we have moved from a manufacturing to a service economy – the manual worker who operated machinery and lifted loads has been replaced by the knowledge worker sitting at a desk all day!

4   Men starting work will usually have participated in sport at school or in higher education, but this often stops on taking up employment or beginning a family due to competing time pressures. The combination of reduced work and leisure time physical activity promotes increased body weight.

5   Chronic overweight and obesity are associated with many diseases that can restrict job opportunities or cause loss of employment due to premature disability. Obesity accounts for 18 million days of sickness absence each year and 30,000 deaths annually. Deaths linked to obesity shorten life by an average of 9 years.

Work and Weight

6   Body weight affects your ability to undertake certain jobs. Being overweight restricts your ability to do job requiring a high degree of fitness or agility.

However, jobs with a lot of regular physical exercise help to burn off the calories and keep down body weight. For instance how often do you see an obese trapeze artist at the circus or skinny Sumo wrestler?

7   Some jobs working with food and drink may encourage overindulgence and becoming overweight.

8   Higher education is associated with increased awareness of personal health and research shows that people with higher qualifications tend to take better care of themselves by not smoking, eating a healthier diet and taking more exercise. Hence it is commonly observed that professionals and managers tend to be healthier and less overweight than less well-qualified workers.

9   A complex mix of work and personal lifestyle influences gives rise to some important effects on body weight. Working overtime may encourage increased body weight due to changed eating habits and reduced leisure time exercise. Also, researchers have reported that obesity may be more prevalent in shift workers.

10   Waist to Hip measurement is suggested as a better marker for body fat distribution. Higher W:H ratios have been reported in male managers than in other male workers and ascribed to the sedentary nature of their work, higher alcohol intake and lower leisure time physical activity.

11   There is no evidence that psychological workload affects body weight. However, comfort eating is very common and many people snack during the day at work. Again overindulgence can lead to becoming overweight.

12   Early life physical fitness predicts later life physical fitness. Those in physically active occupations in early life have a better chance of maintaining body weight in later years.

Fat is not Fit

13   Being overweight has important implications for work fitness. Some specific occupations require a high level of physical fitness, eg, emergency services, and obese persons are at a major disadvantage in achieving the required fitness standards. Exercise testing is sometimes used to see whether an applicant is fit enough to cope with a demanding job.

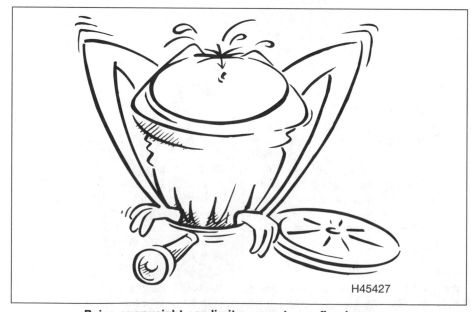

H45427

Being overweight can limit access to confined spaces

14 Some occupations may even be banned for fat people – for instance, obese persons are precluded from commercial diving or working on ships, mainly because they are more likely to have medical problems and are harder to rescue if they do!

15 Being overweight may affect work ability such as climbing ladders or accessing confined spaces. How would you like to be on the ladder, behind the person stuck in the escape hatch because their waist is bigger than hole designed for an average person?

16 Obesity may interfere with the wearing of safety equipment for protection against accidents or harm to health at work. For example unfit overweight people cope less well with tight clothing or wearing a mask.

17 Obese workers are four times more likely to suffer carpal tunnel syndrome, a condition caused by a trapped nerve at the wrist resulting in hand and arm pain.

18 Many occupations have expectations of stereotype images. Obesity can impair self-esteem due to poor body image, and inhibit career advancement and promotion, etc. Anecdotal evidence suggests that some men worry that they may be discriminated against for senior management positions if they are perceived as a health risk in a stressful role. Would you take advice from a 30 stone dietician? (even if they are likely to have had more practice than the 8 stone one!)

Work off the Fat

19 Use your job to develop an exercise routine:
- *Walk or cycle to work.*
- *Park your car at the far side of the car park and walk to the work entrance.*
- *It isn't wasting time – use the time to think!*

20 Vary your job to include more activity:
- *Standing instead of sitting for an hour daily expends additional energy equivalent to 4 lbs (2 kg) of fat per year.*
- *Use the stairs between floors rather than taking the lift.*

21 Plan your work and take the time to walk when you can. Going for a short walk is a great way to take a refreshment break. Exercise has been shown to help you think more clearly – trying to work through without breaks is a mistake!

22 Consider exercise in your longer break times especially if you have a sedentary job:
- *Taking a 20 minute walk each day at a leisurely pace expends additional energy equivalent to 4 lbs (2 kg) of fat per year.*
- *Use the workplace gym or fitness facilities if available.*

23 Try and walk or exercise with friends. This is a great way to relax and develop good and supportive relationships. A shared challenge to lose weight is likely to be more successful and rewarding.

24 Set up a workplace health club:
- *Obtain and distribute information on exercise and healthy eating.*
- *Establish walking paths.*
- *Lobby the canteen to provide healthier choices of foods.*
- *Start a club for those wanting to lose weight.*
- *Ask your employer about health checks at work.*
- *Run competitions to encourage improved fitness and weight loss.*

Further information

25 If you would like to know more, look in the Contacts section at the back of the book, or contact:

The Association for the Study of Obesity
Website: www.aso.org.uk

Fat Facts

- Being very fat or obese is linked to many health problems including heart disease, stroke, diabetes, cancer and arthritis.
- Worldwide there are more than 1 billion overweight adults and at least 300 million are obese.
- Obesity accounts for 2-6% of total health care costs in several developed countries.
- The National Audit Office estimates that obesity costs the NHS £500 million per year and the country up to £7,400 million.
- Over 30,000 deaths per year are caused by obesity in England alone.
- Adult obesity rates have almost quadrupled in the last 25 years.
- 22% of men in UK are obese.
- Overweight men are less likely to be married.
- Fat is less satiating than carbohydrate and protein, but fat increases palatability of diet and encourages over consumption.

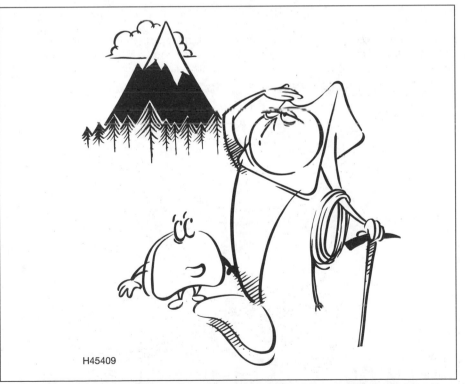

H45409

Try and walk or exercise with friends. A shared challenge to lose weight is likely to be more successful and rewarding

- One hour's brisk walking burns off the calories in a Mars Bar (62.5 grams = 281 kcals).

Regional Facts

- The highest levels of obesity are in the UK regions with lower incomes.

8 Nutrition and football

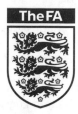

Source: The Official FA Guide to Fitness for Football, published by Hodder Education. See inside rear cover for further information.

1 A healthy diet is one in which the energy intake matches a person's daily demands and over half is provided by carbohydrate-containing foods, less than a third from fat and the remainder from protein.

2 According to the FA, the following snacks are popular amongst athletes. They are high in carbohydrate and relatively low in fat:

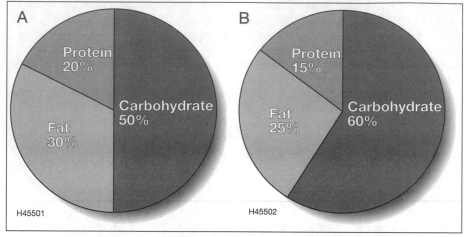

The major food groups and proportional daily requirements

A Normal healthy person (non-sporting)   B Sportsman

- Banana / jam / honey / chocolate spread or peanut butter sandwiches
- Muesli bars or sweetened popcorn
- Fruit cakes, currant buns, scones, American muffins
- Crumpets, bagels, English muffins, Scotch pancakes
- Pop tarts, rusks and cereal
- Jelly cubes and confectionery
- Low-fat rice pudding, bread pudding

3 The FA's nutritionist makes the following recommendations for active sportsmen who need to achieve a low intake of fat as well as a high intake of carbohydrate:

- Base every meal and snack around carbohydrate-rich foods and make sure that these items are the main food on the plate.
- Meats and sauces should be accompaniments to the breads, pasta, rice, potatoes, etc
- Use some reduced fat versions of foods such as milk, spreads, cheeses and yoghurts. Choose lean cuts of meat.
- Grill, poach, bake or microwave food rather than frying or roasting.
- Choose plain cakes, buns and biscuits. These tend to contain less fat than the fancy versions.

Food intake record sheet

Week Commencing . . . .

Monday

Breakfast . . . .

Snack . . . .

Lunch . . . .

Snack . . . .

Dinner . . . .

Supper . . . .

Tuesday

Breakfast . . . .

Snack . . . .

Lunch . . . .

Snack . . . .

Dinner . . . .

Supper . . . .

Food intake record sheet (continued)

Week Commencing . . . .

Wednesday

Breakfast . . . .
Snack . . . .
Lunch . . . .
Snack . . . .
Dinner . . . .
Supper . . . .

Thursday

Breakfast . . . .
Snack . . . .
Lunch . . . .
Snack . . . .
Dinner . . . .
Supper . . . .

Friday

Breakfast . . . .
Snack . . . .
Lunch . . . .
Snack . . . .
Dinner . . . .
Supper . . . .

Saturday

Breakfast . . . .
Snack . . . .
Lunch . . . .
Snack . . . .
Dinner . . . .
Supper . . . .

Sunday

Breakfast . . . .
Snack . . . .
Lunch . . . .
Snack . . . .
Dinner . . . .
Supper . . . .

Log book: Maintenance and Servicing Intervals

Vehicle Type (name) . . . .

Date of First Registration (date of birth) . . . .

Delivery Check Date

Diet		avg cals/day
Alcohol intake		units/week
Smoking		cigs/week
Body Weight		kgs
Exercise		mins/week
Resting Pulse		beats/min
Blood Pressure		/
Blood Cholesterol		mmols/l

1 Month

Diet		avg cals/day
Alcohol intake		units/week
Smoking		cigs/week
Body Weight		kgs
Exercise		mins/week
Resting Pulse		beats/min
Blood Pressure		/
Blood Cholesterol		mmols/l

3 Months

Diet		avg cals/day
Alcohol intake		units/week
Smoking		cigs/week
Body Weight		kgs
Exercise		mins/week
Resting Pulse		beats/min
Blood Pressure		/
Blood Cholesterol		mmols/l

6 Months

Diet		avg cals/day
Alcohol intake		units/week
Smoking		cigs/week
Body Weight		kgs
Exercise		mins/week
Resting Pulse		beats/min
Blood Pressure		/
Blood Cholesterol		mmols/l

9 Months

Diet		avg cals/day
Alcohol intake		units/week
Smoking		cigs/week
Body Weight		kgs
Exercise		mins/week
Resting Pulse		beats/min
Blood Pressure		/
Blood Cholesterol		mmols/l

12 Months

Diet		avg cals/day
Alcohol intake		units/week
Smoking		cigs/week
Body Weight		kgs
Exercise		mins/week
Resting Pulse		beats/min
Blood Pressure		/
Blood Cholesterol		mmols/l

Chapter 5
Going for an MoT

(How a trip to the doctor's can help you to achieve your weight-loss goals)

Contents

1 Assessing your fuel intake

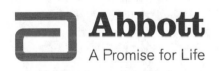

Abbott
A Promise for Life

1 Obesity is one of the fastest growing medical conditions in the UK. In 1980, only 6% of men were clinically obese. Now, as many as 21% of UK men fit into the obese category[1].

2 There are a number of possible reasons.

• Firstly, we have all become less active. The birth of the computer age has meant that we can all enjoy a wide variety of home-based entertainment, in the comfort of our armchairs. The popularity of digital television, DVDs, video game consoles and the internet has resulted in fewer people taking regular exercise. This means that, on average, people are now burning fewer calories than ever.

• Secondly, high-fat convenience foods such as pizzas, burgers, chips and deep-fried chicken meals have become extremely popular. These foods are now part of the nation's staple diet, and their cheap, super-size portions mean that, on average, people are now consuming more calories than ever.

3 Bearing this in mind, it is not difficult to understand why so many people are now overweight.

4 The simple facts are:

• If you take in more calories than your body needs, you will put on weight. Conversely:

• If your body uses up more calories than you take in, you will lose weight.

5 Put simply, a calorie is the amount of energy that is contained within a food. The higher the number of calories, the more energy that is locked away inside it.

6 Unfortunately, by judging portion size alone, it is very difficult to tell how many calories a particular food contains. Certain foods (eg, chocolate) are very calorie-dense, meaning that even a small portion is very high in calories. Other foods (eg, vegetables) are calorie-sparse, meaning that even large portions are not likely to result in substantial weight gain.

Strange but true
There are more calories in a small (50 gram) bar of chocolate than there are in three bananas.

---

7 To get a true picture of the number of calories in a food, it is important to read the food's nutrition label.

8 This will not only provide information about the calorific value of 100ml/100g of the food (or a typical serving size), but will also usually tell you:

• *The amount of protein (in grams).*
• *The amount of sugaring and non-sugaring carbohydrates (in grams).*
• *The amount of saturated and unsaturated fat (in grams).*
• *The amount of fibre (in grams).*
• *The amount of salt [sodium] (in grams).*

Calculate your body mass index (BMI)

This is simply your weight in kilograms, divided by the square of your height in metres:

$$\frac{\text{Weight (kg)}}{\text{Height (m)}^2}$$

Example:

Joe weighs 70.5 kg, and is 1.82 m tall. His BMI is therefore:

$$\frac{70.5}{1.82 \times 1.82} = \frac{70.5}{3.3124} = 21.3$$

What the results mean

BMI	Weight Status
Below 18.5	Underweight
18.6 to 24.9	Normal
25.0 to 29.9	Overweight
30.0 and above	Obese

2 The importance of regular maintenance checks

1 If you are prone to putting on weight, you should make regular checks to ensure that your weight is not getting out of hand. Even losing small amounts of weight can have a significant positive impact on your overall health. For example, losing some excess weight will substantially reduce your chance of contracting cancer and heart disease[2].

2 If you think you will find it difficult to lose weight on your own, your doctor is ready, willing and able to help you achieve your weight-loss goals. When you visit your doctor for the first time, he or she will probably run a series of tests. These tests are rather like an MoT, as they tell the doctor all he needs to know about your excess fat levels and the way they are affecting your overall health.

3 Using the results of your MoT, the doctor will be able to:

- Assess how much weight you need to lose.
- Suggest a sensible weight-loss rate (usually around 0.5 to 1 kg (1 to 2 lbs) per week).
- Help with a plan of action to help you lose weight (eg, balanced diet, exercise regime, weight-loss medication).

4 Your doctor or practice nurse will be able to provide a number of weight-loss services. The exact services offered will vary from practice to practice, but most doctors can provide:

- A series of tests to make sure that your weight gain has not caused an underlying condition such as diabetes.
- A healthy eating plan.
- A sensible exercise regimen.
- Expert advice and support.
- Anti-obesity drug treatment.

3 To get the most from your visit, follow a few simple rules

Make weight loss the sole reason for seeing your doctor

1 Losing weight is an important clinical issue. If you only mention it at the end of a consultation about something else, your doctor may mistakenly believe that you are not committed to losing your excess weight. Reducing obesity is a priority for the NHS, so you should give your doctor enough time to be able to discuss your weight loss in detail.

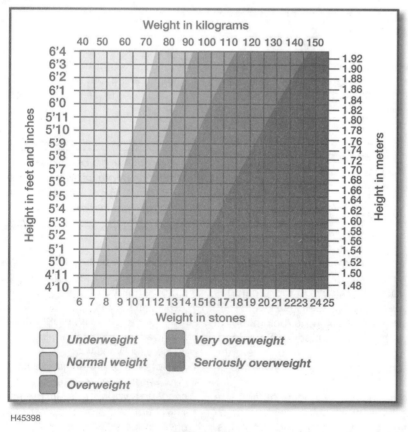

H45398

BMI graph

This applies to both adult men and women, but not sportspeople as muscle is heavier than fat

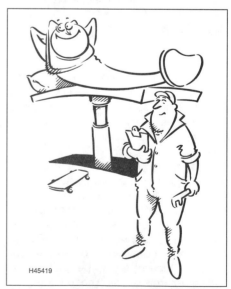

H45419

Your doctor will assess how weight is affecting your overall health

Show your doctor that you are serious about losing weight

2 Losing weight needs a commitment from you too. Explain that you are determined to lose weight, and that you fully understand that this will entail sensible eating and regular exercise. You could also take this opportunity to ask about the various treatment options which will help to aid the weight-loss process.

Tell your doctor about your previous weight-loss experiences

3 You need to be totally honest with your doctor, in order to receive the advice and support that is right for you. Openly describe your eating habits and current levels of physical activity, and tell your doctor about any previous weight-loss attempts. It is important for him to understand why these attempts failed, so that you are successful this time.

Tell your doctor or practice nurse about how being fat is making you feel

4 Although it may seem difficult at first, it will help your doctor or nurse if you could explain how being fat makes you feel. Be as open and as honest as you can. Don't just describe the physical repercussions (eg, shortness of breath, frequent tiredness), also try to describe how you feel on an emotional level (eg, does your weight problem leave you feeling depressed, do you 'comfort eat'?).

4 Visiting an 'obesity bodyshop'

1 Some practices also offer dedicated weight-loss clinics. This type of clinic provides frequent motivation and continuous advice.
2 Clinics usually last around 20-30 minutes and are held at fortnightly intervals. The person who runs the clinic may be your doctor or your practice nurse.
3 The itinerary is designed to be educational and varied, and will help to keep you motivated as you strive to lose your excess weight. You should be prepared to commit to attending the clinic for at least one year.
4 Activities at these weight-loss clinics may include:

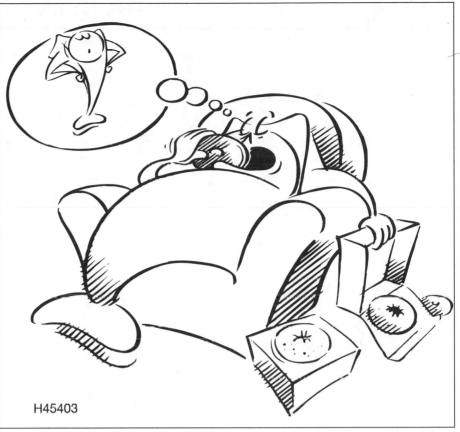

H45403

Does your weight problem make you comfort eat?

- *Thinking about the main reasons why you have become overweight.*
- *Thinking about how losing weight will improve your health and quality of life.*
- *Monitoring food intake and physical activity.*
- *Developing a basic understanding of nutrients and food groups.*
- *Learning techniques for staying in control when you are eating out.*
- *Reading and interpreting food labels to help identify healthy and unhealthy foods.*
- *Identifying your trigger foods (foods that you have trouble stopping eating) and planning to avoid them.*
- *Developing an appropriate programme for increase in physical activities.*

5 Getting a jump start

1 If you are finding it difficult to lose weight, your doctor can also prescribe special weight-loss medications.
2 There are currently two medications that can help to boost your weight loss attempts. Both of these medications must be taken alongside a sensible diet and exercise programme, and are only suitable if your BMI is more than 27 and if you have other obesity-related conditions, or if your BMI is greater than 30.
3 These two medications are called sibutramine and orlistat.
- Sibutramine works by helping you learn to eat less. You are therefore able to eat smaller meal portions without feeling hungry. When used in conjunction with a low-calorie diet and exercise programme, studies have shown that most people on sibutramine achieve initial weight losses of at least 5-10% (eg, a minimum of 5-10 kg in a 100 kg man)[3].
- Orlistat impedes absorbtion of up to a third of the fat you take in from your diet[4]. It is important that people on orlistat stick to a low-fat diet.
4 If you feel that you would benefit from taking either of these medications, you should visit your doctor.

References

Written by Dr David Haslam

1 National Audit Office. Tackling Obesity in England. Report by the Comptroller and Auditor General, HC 220, Session 2001-2001.

2 Haslam DW. Obesity - the scale of the problem. General Practitioner July 2001; pp 31-32.

3 James WPT, Astrup A, Finer N et al. Effect of sibutramine on weight maintenance after weight loss: a randomized trial. Lancet 2000; 356: 2119-2125.

4 Sjöström L, Torgerson JS, Hauptman J et al. Xenical in the prevention of diabetes in obese subjects: a landmark study. Abstract presented at the 9th International Congress on Obesity, São Paulo, Brazil, 24-29 August 2002.

Chapter 6
Avoidable medical problems

Contents

1 Health and more general impacts

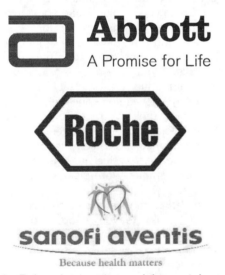

1 Being obese or overweight can take a terrible toll on your health. Almost every man who is obese develops weight-related symptoms by his 40th birthday. Most need medical treatment for a disease caused by their obesity by the age of 60 years[1]. And obesity kills around 30,000 people each year[2]. Indeed, young men with BMI of 30 are about 50% more likely to die early than someone with a healthy weight. Mature men with BMI of 35 are more than twice as likely to die early as their leaner counterparts[3]. (See Chapter 5 for BMI calculation.)

2 Excess weight kills because it causes or aggravates many diseases. For instance, obesity causes about a quarter of cases of hypertension (dangerously high blood pressure), strokes and type II diabetes. It causes around a fifth of cases of angina and gout as well as one in six heart attacks and gall bladder problems[4]. Being overweight can undermine self-confidence and can lead to depression and other psychological problems. The clichéd idea of a merry fat man is often a myth. This Section looks at three of the most common problems associated with obesity.

Heart disease and strokes

3 Cardiovascular disease – mainly heart disease and strokes – kills more people than anything else. Heart disease accounts for half of cardiovascular deaths, killing more than one in five men[5]. Many more men live with the symptoms of heart disease – such as the crippling pain of angina. Half of all 40-year-old men will develop heart disease sometime during the rest of their life[6].

4 The most common form of heart disease arises when fatty deposits – known as atherosclerotic plaques – build up on the walls of the blood vessels supplying the heart. These plaques narrow the blood vessels. So the supply of oxygen and nutrients to the heart muscles falls. Angina signals that the heart is not getting enough oxygen and forces sufferers to slow down, which re-balances supply and demand.

5 These plaques can rupture, causing their contents to flood into the blood stream triggering a blood clot which further reduces or totally blocks the blood supply to the heart, leading to a heart attack (also called a myocardial infarction). That's why many men who are at high risk take an aspirin a day to keep the cardiologist away. At low doses, aspirin – lower than you'd take for a headache – makes the blood less likely to clot. But don't do this without talking to your doctor first: it isn't right for everyone.

6 There are two types of stroke, both of which can cause death and disability, and account for about a quarter of deaths from cardiovascular disease[7]. Like heart attacks, 'ischaemic' strokes, which account for 85 per cent of strokes, arise when fatty plaques build up, this time in the blood vessels supplying the brain. If these plaques rupture, the blood clot can starve areas of the brain of oxygen and nutrients, so the brain cells die. The other type, 'haemorrhagic' strokes, occur when blood vessels supplying the brain burst, causing blood to leak into the brain and clot, destroying brain cells.

7 Numerous factors contribute to heart disease and ischaemic strokes. You can't do anything about some of these risk factors – such as your age, being male or carrying genes linked to heart disease. But you can change others, such as being overweight (in particular having a large waist size), not exercising or smoking. Your doctor can help with still others such as high levels of cholesterol in your blood, diabetes and hypertension[8]. As we'll see later in the Section many of these risk factors cluster together in susceptible individuals.

8 Having a large waist size is especially

dangerous. Your body stores fat either under the skin or within your gut (known as visceral fat). Recently, doctors showed just how dangerous a large waist really is. A major international study – called INTERHEART – found that abnormal levels of cholesterol and fats in the blood accounted for about half the risk of suffering a heart attack; high blood pressure for 30% and a large waist size for the remaining 20%[9].

Type II diabetes

9   Add sugar to your tea and coffee and you're adding a form of carbohydrate: sucrose. The body rapidly absorbs sucrose, which it breaks down into glucose which your cells use as fuel. Your body carefully controls blood glucose levels to balance supply and demand using a complex network of chemical signals. A hormone, called insulin, produced by your pancreas (a gland near your liver) is one of the most important of these signals. Insulin tells cells to increase the amount of sugar they take up from your blood.

10 Insulin binds to receptors on cells. Think of the receptor as the ignition on your car and insulin as the key. Insulin fits into the receptor and switches on the cell's biological engines. The binding is exact, just like the key in the lock. Insulin's binding allows glucose to pass from the blood into the cell. The cell either uses glucose for energy or, in the case of liver or muscle cells, stores it (as glycogen). In many obese men, the system develops a fault, and the cells *resist* the action of insulin, so the sugar in the blood is left floating around with nowhere to go. At first the body overcomes this, by sending for re-inforcements and producing more insulin to overcome the resistance, so the sugar level stays normal. After a while, however, the system becomes overloaded, and the body can no longer cope with the vast amount of insulin required, and the inevitable result is a raised blood sugar, and eventually diabetes.

11 So diabetes arises when this system goes wrong, and levels of sugar in the blood become too high. Over time, high blood sugar levels can lead to serious conditions including ulcers on your feet and even amputations, blindness, kidney damage, strokes and heart attacks.

Doctors can easily identify these changes in the blood at a very early stage, and prevent the disastrous conditions which may otherwise occur, but he's not a magician, and he can't do this unless you go and see him. Doctors often diagnose type II diabetes only when the person develops heart disease or another complication. Many men with type II diabetes may not develop the classic signs of diabetes, such as blurred visions, extreme thirst or infections you can't shake off. There are well over 1,000,000 undiagnosed diabeteics in this country, so, if you are overweight you should be checked for diabetes.

12 These complications make diabetes a killer. A man who weighs 40% more than the ideal is more than five times more likely to die from diabetes than a man of healthy weight[10]. Deaths from heart disease are five times more common among people with diabetes than in healthy men. Stroke is up to three times more common among men with diabetes[11]. Because of these complications, life expectancy is up to 10 years shorter among men with type II diabetes compared to the general population[12].

13 There are two types of diabetes. A faulty immune system causes the classic type I diabetes, which usually arises during childhood. The immune system evolved to repel bacterial, viral and other infections. Occasionally, these immune cells can turn against our body causing so-called autoimmune diseases. In type I diabetes, the immune system destroys the cells that produce insulin. People with type I diabetes need regular injections to replace the insulin that should be produced by the pancreas.

14 Some 1.3 million adults in the UK have type II diabetes[13], making it far more common than the autoimmune form. Type II diabetes tends to emerge in middle-age, but the obesity epidemic means that a growing number of children now develop the condition.

15 Diets high in sugar and refined carbohydrate, such as white bread, biscuits, cakes, rice and potatoes, mean that we need to produce more insulin to control blood sugar levels. Lack of exercise reduces the amount of sugar our muscles and other cells take from the blood. Glucose is the body's petrol; it's fuel, and just like a car, the more you

move the more fuel you need. Keep your car in the drive and you don't fill up very often. Sitting quietly for a couple of hours uses around 150 kcal, while walking 6 miles in two hours uses 500 kcal. (The difference is about the same as three slices of bread and butter[14].) A calorie dense diet and a sedentary lifestyle contribute to obesity. Being overweight means there are more cells and, in some people, not enough insulin to ensure they all work properly. Once again, doctors now recognise that visceral fat – reflected in a large waist size – is linked to a particularly high risk of developing diabetes. Indeed, many men from some ethnic minorities – such as those whose family came from India – have an even greater risk of developing diabetes, even though by Caucasian standards they may be not particularly obese.

Metabolic syndrome

16 Forget what your maths teacher told you. Sometimes 2 plus 2 can equal five. If you have one risk factor for heart disease and then develop another, the risks don't just add together. For example, if you have hypertension your risk of suffering a heart attack is three times higher than someone with normal blood pressure. If you have both raised serum cholesterol and hypertension you are nine times more likely to develop heart disease than the average man. If you also smoke, your risk is 16 fold higher[15].

17 In 1988, an American researcher called Gerald Reaven recognised that having a large amount of visceral fat, in conjunction with other risk factors, dramatically increased the risk of developing heart disease and other conditions[16]. Today, doctors call this cluster of risk factors the metabolic syndrome. If you have three or more at of the following you have the metabolic syndrome:

• Waist circumference of at least 40 inches (102 cm). This should not be measured where the waistband of your trousers sits but higher up around the level of your belly button where your waistline is at its largest.
• Triglycerides over 150 mg/dl (1.7 mmol/l). Triglycerides are a type of fat in your blood. Like the better known low-density lipoprotein (LDL; remember L for lethal) high levels of

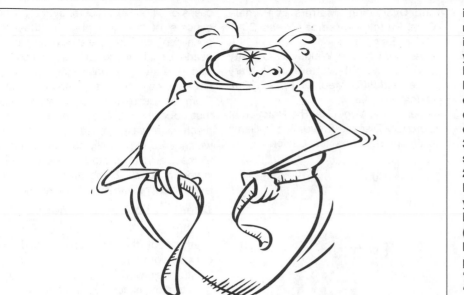

Waist circumference should be measured around the level of your belly button where your waistline is at its largest

triglycerides increase your risk of developing heart disease.

- Levels of high-density lipoprotein (HDL) cholesterol under 40 mg/dl (1.0 mmol/l). HDL is the good fat – remember H for healthy. HDL carries cholesterol from your tissue to your liver, where it is destroyed.
- Blood pressure over 130/80 mmHg.
- A level of glucose in your blood while fasting over 110 mg/dl (6.11 mmol/l).

18 To find out your level of the last four in this list, you need to enlist the help of your GP. But if you've piled on the inches around the gut it is a good idea to get them checked.

Cancer

19 Diet plays an important role in determining your risk of developing cancer. Eating a healthy diet – one high in fruit and vegetables and low in fat, for example – reduces your risk of dying from cancer by about a third. Obesity also directly contributes to cancer. Experts believe that obesity probably causes about 3% of cancers in European men. Excess weight causes about 7% of all cancer deaths among non-smokers[17]. In comparison, smoking causes just under two in every five (36%) cancers in men.[18] Quitting smoking, eating a healthy diet and staying at a

healthy weight can dramatically reduce your chances of succumbing to cancer.

Losing weight

20 Clearly, losing excess weight is good for your health, but it's important to be realistic. A weight loss of around 2.5 kg

in the first four weeks is practical for most men; aim to lose 5% of your weight in the first three months and 10% over a year[19]. Although it doesn't sound much, losing 10% of your weight can make a big difference to your health. For example, your risk of dying prematurely declines by more than 20%. Your risk of death from diabetes falls by at least 30%[20]. Losing about a kilo of weight can shrink your waist band by about 1 cm.

21 A 10% fall in weight also reduces blood pressure and helps cut fat levels in your blood. For instance, your diastolic blood pressure may fall by 20 mmHg. (Diastolic is the blood pressure when the heart relaxes between beats.) If your blood pressure is 125 over 80, the 80 is your 'diastolic' pressure; the 125 is your 'systolic' (the pressure when the heart contracts). Levels of LDL-cholesterol (the dangerous fat) fall by 15%. Levels of HDL-cholesterol (the good fat;) rise by 8%[21].

22 To put these change in context, a 1 mmHg fall in diastolic blood pressure reduces the risk of death by between 2% and 4%. A 1.5 mg/dl decline in LDL-C reduces mortality by between 1 and 1.5%. A 0.5 mg/dl increase in HDL-C also reduces the risk of death by between 1 and 1.5%[22]. In other words, losing weight doesn't just make you look and feel better, it could save your life.

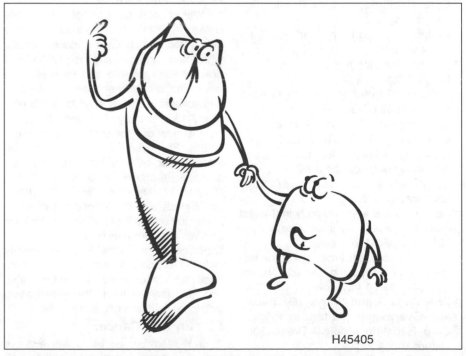

Losing weight is good for your health, but it's important to be realistic

References

1 Chambers R and Wakley G Obesity and Overweight Matters in Primary Care Radcliffe Medical Press 2002 Oxford page 11.

2 National Audit Commission Tackling Obesity in England 2001 p16.

3 National Audit Commission Tackling Obesity in England 2001 p16.

4 Chambers R and Wakley G Obesity and Overweight Matters in Primary Care Radcliffe Medical Press 2002 Oxford table 1.4.

5 www.heartstats.org p12.

6 Liu JLY, Maniadakis, Gray A et al The economic burden of coronary heart disease in the UK Heart 2002;88:597

7 www.heartstats.org p12.

8 Gaw A, Lindsay GM and Shepherd J Cardiovascular disease: atherosclerosis in Tomlinson S, Heagerty AM and Weetman AP eds Mechanisms of Disease: An Introduction To Clinical Science Cambridge University Press first edition 1997 p257.

9 Yusuf S, Hawken S, Ôunpuu S et al Effect of potentially modifiable risk factors associated with myocardial infarction in 52 countries (the INTERHEART study): case-control study Lancet 2004; 364: p937–52.

10 Chambers R and Wakley G Obesity and Overweight Matters in Primary Care Radcliffe Medical Press 2002 Oxford page 12.

11 National Service Framework (NFS) for Diabetes p10.

12 NSF for Diabetes p10.

13 NSF for Diabetes p9.

14 Wiseman G Nutrition & Health Taylor & Francis 2002 p5-6.

15 Betteridge DJ and Morrell JM Clinicians' Guide to Lipids and Coronary Heart Disease Second edition Arnold, London 2003 p38.

16 http://www.cacr.ca/news/2000/0009reaven.htm.

17 Peto J Cancer epidemiology in the last century and the next decade Nature 2001;411:390-1 in green.

18 Peto J Cancer epidemiology in the last century and the next decade Nature 2001;411:390-1 in yellow.

19 Chambers R and Wakley G Obesity and Overweight Matters in Primary Care Radcliffe Medical Press 2002 Oxford Box 4.2.

20 Chambers R and Wakley G Obesity and Overweight Matters in Primary Care Radcliffe Medical Press 2002 Oxford Box 4.3.

21 Chambers R and Wakley G Obesity and Overweight Matters in Primary Care Radcliffe Medical Press 2002 Oxford Box 4.3.

22 Miller M and Vogel RA The Practice of Coronary Disease Prevention Williams & Wilkins Baltimore first edition p5.

2 Taking the taboo out of poo

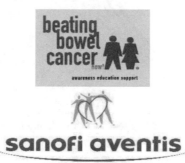

This section has been developed by the national charity Beating Bowel Cancer and supported by an unrestricted educational grant from sanofi-aventis. Introduction from media dietician Lyndel Costain, BSc, RD.

Obesity and Health

1 Weight can be one of life's more challenging and sensitive issues. While you don't need to look like an Adonis (despite what media images suggest) to be fit, it does make sense to aim to keep to a weight that is healthy and feels comfortable and achievable. The fact is that there's now a very powerful body of research that spells out just how dangerous obesity is for our health. For example, a report by the National Audit Office concluded that, on average, it shaves nine years off our lifespan. Studies have also revealed that obesity increases the risk of type II diabetes in men by up to 42 times, and 14 per cent of male cancers can be attributed to it. Other health problems linked to obesity include heart disease and strokes, snoring, back pain, osteoarthritis, reduced sex drive and fertility, asthma, breathlessness, gallstones, hiatus hernia and low mood.

Obesity and Cancer

2 In Western Europe, being overweight or obese accounts for an estimated 1 in 10 cases of all bowel cancers, over a third of cancers of the oesophagus (the tube connecting the mouth and stomach), and a quarter of kidney and gall bladder cancers. Cancer is a very complex disease, and it's not yet clear why obesity has this effect. From what researchers do know, it seems that obesity could increase risk in mechanical ways; for example, too much weight around the belly causes damaging stomach acid reflux into the oesophagus; or in hormonal ways by abnormally increasing levels of cell growth-stimulating hormones.

Obesity and Bowel cancer

3 Studies indicate that obese men have nearly double the risk of developing bowel cancer compared to men who are a healthy weight. This may be because men tend to store excess body fat around their waist or abdomen – the classic 'belly' syndrome. Too much abdominal fat can lead to a condition called 'insulin resistance' which causes the body to produce higher and higher amounts of insulin and other insulin-like growth factors. This, it is believed, stimulates bowel cells to divide more rapidly, and increases the risk of the random cell damage that can lead to cancer. Other studies suggest that high levels of a hormone called leptin may also play a role.

4 Bowel cancer risk is also linked to eating a lot of red meat and too few fibre-rich whole grains, fruit and vegetables, and not being active. These diet and lifestyle habits are also common risk factors for gaining weight, so there is a lot of overlap. Regular physical activity is worth special mention as it can not only help you get to and/or keep to a healthier weight but helps regulate levels of insulin and other hormones in the blood. Physical activity may also speed the passage of carcinogens (cancer causing agents) from the body so reducing the amount of time they can spend in contact with the lining of the bowel.

So, do you really have anything to worry about?

5 Well, the facts suggest that you do:
- Bowel cancer is the second most deadly cancer in the UK – only lung cancer kills more people.
- Around 35,600 people are diagnosed with the disease each year and over 45% will die as a result.
- Bowel cancer affects men and women almost equally, and more men will die

from it. Part of the reason is late diagnosis.

- In the league table of the most common male cancers, bowel cancer comes in at third place after cancer of skin and prostate.

Look on the bright side

6 Shocking statistics, yes, But, the good news is that armed with these facts, you are now in a position to take action and reduce your risk. By taking simple steps to look after yourself, you will not only feel and look better but will also know that you are doing all you can to protect yourself from a number of serious health problems such as bowel cancer.

7 Bowel cancer is one of the most curable cancers if caught early enough. It is estimated that around 90% of cases could be treated successfully if caught at an early stage.

8 Getting over your embarrassment could help to save your life. Many people are too embarrassed to discuss their symptoms and delay seeking medical advice. It is vital to look out for possible symptoms and have them investigated (by a health professional such as your GP) if they persist (see symptom information below)

9 There are lots of common conditions that could cause changes in the workings of the bowels, pain and bleeding from the bottom. In most cases, it won't be cancer.

Your risk increases if there is bowel cancer in the family, but diet and smoking are among the main culprits.

What is bowel cancer?

10 The large bowel is a question-mark-shaped tube of muscle – about four feet long – which runs from the appendix, via the colon, to the rectum. Bowel cancer is cancer of any part of this tube. If it is not treated, it will increase in size and may cause a blockage, or it can ulcerate, leading to blood loss and anaemia.

11 Most cancers start with wart-like growths known as polyps on the wall of the gut. Polyps are very common as we get older – one in ten people over 60 have them. However, most polyps do not turn into cancer. If potentially cancerous polyps can be found at an early stage, they can be removed painlessly without the need for an operation.

Eating healthily

12 So, we know that experts now believe that our eating habits can influence the risk of developing cancer, particularly of the bowel, stomach, mouth, throat, oesophagus and pancreas. But as yet we don't fully understand which parts of our diet constitute a risk factor and which could be protective. The effect of diet on cancer risk may also be influenced by genes. All these areas are currently being researched to increase our understanding and to help more people to prevent cases in the future.

13 However, what is certain is that choosing to eat healthily is something that everyone can do to help reduce their risk of developing cancer.

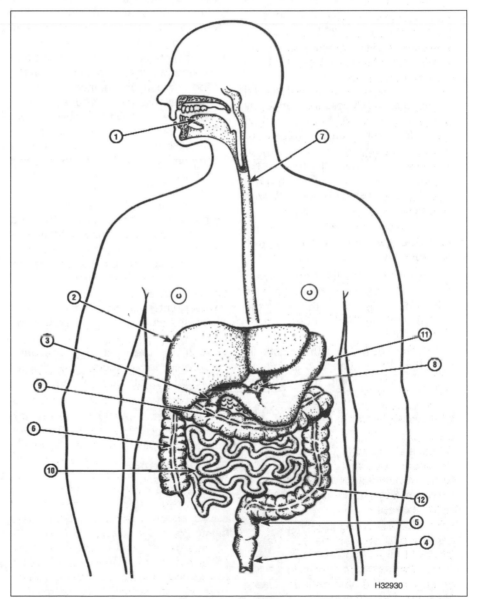

The digestive system

1 *Tongue*	5 *Caecum*	9 *Transverse colon*
2 *Liver*	6 *Ascending colon*	10 *Small intestine*
3 *Duodenum*	7 *Oesophagus*	11 *Stomach*
4 *Rectum*	8 *Pancreas*	12 *Descending colon*

H32930

14 Ideally, healthy eating habits should start early – in our childhood. But don't worry, it's never too late to start eating a healthy, balanced diet. The basic checklist includes:

- *Plenty of fruit and vegetables.*
- *Foods high in fibre.*
- *Starchy foods such as potatoes, pasta and rice.*
- *Reduce your intake of fat and salt.*
- *Minimise the amount of processed and red meats in your diet.*

15 More generally, it is always a good idea to get into a healthy eating 'pattern'. It is worth keeping in mind that:

- Small meals taken regularly are better for you than long periods without food, followed by a heavy meal.
- Large, rich meals late at night should be avoided if at all possible, especially for older people. A midday cooked meal is more easily digested.
  - Make sure that you drink plenty of fluids – at least one and a half litres a day and more if the weather is hot – especially if you should become ill with an infection.

The digestive system: how does it work?

16 From the moment food enters your mouth, until it leaves your body, it makes an incredible journey through the digestive system. So how does it really work?

- Your tastebuds (all 10,000) are actually nerve-endings which send signals to your brain – meaning that you can experience different taste sensations such as salt, sweet or bitter.
- Your teeth grind the food into digestible pieces.
- Saliva moistens the food so that it doesn't scrape your digestive tract on the way down.
- Once you've swallowed your food, it's carried down the oesophagus into your stomach.
- Your stomach walls churns the food up to make sure it's mixed with your acidic digestive juices.
- Once liquefied into a mixture called chyme, it is squirted through a small hole into your small intestine.
- Your pancreas releases an alkaline and enzymes which help to break down the food's carbohydrates, fat and protein.
- Your gall bladder produces bile to make sure that any fat is broken down.
- The food is now reduced down to tiny particles which can be absorbed through the walls of your small intestine.
- The nutrients from your food are carried into your blood stream.
- Any nutrients that can't be absorbed end up in the small intestine – including fibre, which has certain components that can't be absorbed by the human body.
- Finally, anything left over is classed as waste matter, stored in the rectum and released as a stool – the end of the journey.

17 A high fibre diet is particularly recognised for reducing the risk of constipation, irritable bowel syndrome and bowel cancer. Fibre is indigestible plant material such as cellulose, lignin and pectin, which is found in fruits, vegetables, grains and beans.

18 There are two types of fibre – soluble and insoluble. Fibre provides bulk to your food, helps it pass easily through the gut and also retains water (making us feel full and therefore we eat less).

19 Reports suggest that we should be eating 18g of fibre each day – yet most of us probably eat much less (around 10-12g). To give a couple of examples, a banana contains 1.8g, as does 1 slice of wholemeal toast.

20 When increasing your fibre intake, start slowly and build up to the recommended level. Here are some tips:

- Replace lower fibre foods with high fibre foods (see chart below), eg, choose whole grain breads and cereals.
- Eat vegetables and fruit raw whenever possible.
- Steam or stir-fry vegetables if you need to cook them – boiling can cause up to one half of the fibre to be lost in the water.
- Replace fruit or vegetable juice with the whole fruit – fruit skin and membranes are a particularly good source of fibre.
- Start your day with a bowl of high-fibre cereal (5g of fibre or more per serving). Add fresh fruit or sprinkle with wheat germ or bran for an easy way to build up fibre intake.
- Eat only whole grain products.

HIGH FIBRE FOOD	LOWER FIBRE FOOD
Whole grain breads, eg, 100% whole wheat, cracked wheat, multigrain, pumpernickel or dark rye	White bread
Whole grain cereal containing bran, oatmeal, barley, bulgar, cracked wheat; also Shredded Wheat, multigrain or granola cereals	Refined cereals
Whole grain flours, eg, whole wheat, rye, graham (eg, biscuits, muffins)	Foods made with white flour
Whole grain pastas, brown rice or wild rice	Refined pastas, instant or polished rice
Fresh fruits and veg	Fruit juice
Salads (with variety of raw vegetables)	Plain lettuce salads
Baked beans, cooked lentils, split peas	Meat, fish; poultry
Nuts, popcorn, seeds, dried fruit	Crisps, other snacks

Red and processed meat

21 There are many British food traditions which fuel our ongoing love-affair with red meat – think Sunday roast, shepherd's pie, steak and kidney pie. Red meat is a good source of protein, vitamins, minerals and iron – all important components of a healthy diet.
22 However, we shouldn't eat too much of it – as there is some evidence to suggest that eating lots of red meat (pork, lamb and beef), processed meat (eg, sausages, burgers and pies) and cured meat (eg, bacon and ham) is a risk factor for bowel cancer. These foods are also often high in fat. So, including some red meat in your diet is fine, but try to substitute it where possible with alternative sources of protein like chicken, turkey or fish.

Adding colour to your life

23 To make healthy eating easier and more enjoyable, experts suggest following the traffic light rule: RED, AMBER, GREEN. For example, make sure that you have enough variety in your diet and try to eat a mixture of fruit and vegetables that are different colours every day to ensure that you get the maximum nutritional benefit. Why not try:
• *Beetroot, carrots and spinach.*
• *Red peppers, oranges and broccoli.*
• *Tomatoes, pumpkin and peas.*
• *Strawberries, orange pepper and courgette.*

Exercise for life

24 Recent research has found compelling evidence that regular exercise could cut the risk of developing bowel cancer by 50%. To help reduce the risk of cancer, people should aim for 30 minutes of moderate intensity physical activity at least three times a week. Get physical with the following bite-size exercise tips:
• *Wash and wax your car.*
• *Take the dog for a walk.*
• *Get out in the garden – do your weeding or rake the leaves.*
• *Walk or cycle to work rather than get in the car again.*
• *Go for a bike ride with your family or friends.*
• *Go for a swim.*
• *Take the stairs rather than the lift at work or in the shopping centre.*

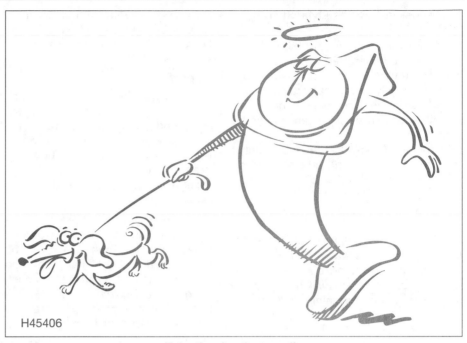

H45406

Take the dog for a walk

• *Roll your sleeves up and get dirty with the housework – washing the windows or doing the vacuuming can be quite physical.*

Don't sit on your symptoms

Common symptoms

25 It may sound unpleasant – but keeping a check on your bowel habits is the best way of making sure you spot any symptoms of bowel cancer in the early stages. The most common symptoms are change of bowel habit and rectal bleeding. However, these are also common in people who don't have cancer. The facts show that:
• Nearly 20% of us experience bleeding from the bottom each year.
• Over a third of us experience constipation or diarrhoea at some point in our lives.
26 As mentioned earlier, there are lots of common conditions that could cause changes in the workings of the bowels, pain and bleeding from the bottom. In most cases, it won't be cancer.

Early detection gives the best protection, so know your bum chum.

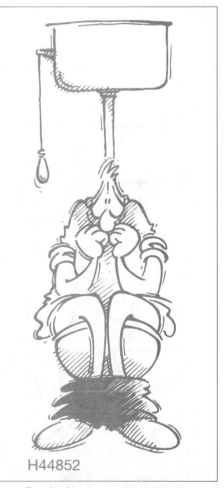

H44852

Don't sit on your symptoms

Higher risk symptoms – 'watch and wait'

27 If you have any of the higher risk symptoms outlined below, it is safe to 'watch and wait' for up to six weeks. But if they persist, you should get advice from your GP and ask about the possibility of further investigation at your local hospital.

28 Change of bowel habit (especially important if you also have bleeding) – a recent, persistent change of bowel habit to looser, more diarrhoea-like motions, going to the toilet or trying to 'go' more often

29 Rectal bleeding – look out for rectal bleeding that persists with no reason. For example, bleeding can be due to piles – but if so you will have other symptoms such as straining with hard stools, a sore bottom, lumps and itching. If you are over 60, piles could be hiding more serious symptoms, so it is especially important to get this investigated

Other high risk symptoms and signs

- Unexplained anaemia, found by your GP.
- A lump or mass in your abdomen, felt by your GP.

- Persistent, severe abdominal pain which has come on recently for the first time (especially in older people).

The perfect poo

Most healthy adults need to empty their bowels about twice a day. If you are healthy and eating enough fibre, the stool should be firm, light brown in colour, and float in the toilet bowl. An average stool is 75% water. The remainder is made up of fibre, dead cells and bacteria.

What your poo says about you

- Stinking stools: can be a sign of poor digestion and food stagnation in the large intestine. Try to eat more high fibre foods to help 'push' food through the digestive system.
- Pebble-dash – your liver may be congested. Foods that enrich the liver include cauliflower, cabbage, broccoli, garlic.
- Loose and runny stools – this may be a sign that you do not have enough fibre in your diet. Check-out the list of high fibre foods in the table above. Diarrohea-like stools for over 6 weeks could be a sign or something more serious like bowel cancer so do visit

your GP if your toilet habits are out of character.

Don't die of embarrassment – visit your GP without delay if you've been experiencing symptoms for a period of around six weeks

Is there anything else I need to know about bowel cancer?

Family history

30 If you ask around in your family, you may well find someone who has had bowel cancer. While bowel cancer can in some cases be put down to genetics, family history doesn't necessarily mean that you are going to get it. In general, the closer the relatives are to you (eg, brother, sister, mother, father or child) and the younger they were diagnosed, the more you need to get it checked out.

31 The following is a guide to the action you may need to take depending on your family history:

- One close relative under 45 affected – talk to your GP about screening in your area. It is usually recommended 10 years before the age at which your relative developed the disease.

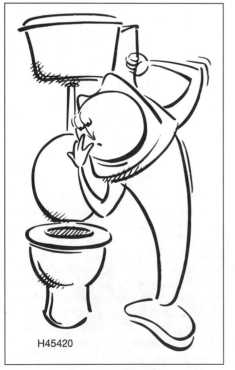

H45420

The perfect poo

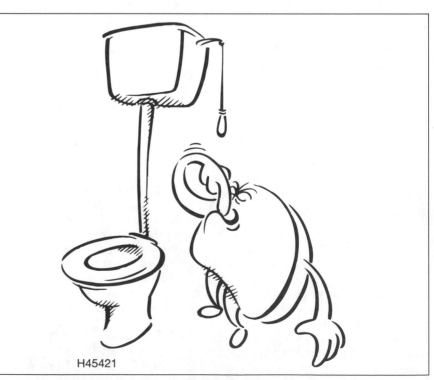

H45421

The smell could be a sign of poor digestion and food stagnation in the gut

- Two or more close relatives from the same side of the family – the younger those relatives, the more need there is for you to discuss screening with your GP.
- Less strong family history (such as a grandparent who died in their 70s) – you are probably not at an increased risk. However, do talk to your GP if you are worried.

Further information

32 If you would like to know more, look in the Contacts section at the back of the book, or contact:

Beating Bowel Cancer

The charity also has a range of free factsheets covering specific topics relating to bowel cancer, such as Diet for Bowel Cancer Patients, Treatment Choices and Bowel Cancer and Genetics and Bowel Cancer Screening.

Current information available:

- *Bowel cancer: The Bottom Line* (booklet).
- *Don't Sit on Your Symptoms* (leaflet).
- *Treating Bowel Cancer: Your Choices* (booklet).
- *Dietary Advice for Bowel Cancer Patients* (leaflet).

Tel: 020 8892 5256
e-mail: Info@beatingbowelcancer.org
Website: www.beatingbowelcancer.org

Did you know?

- In an average lifetime your gut will take in 65 tonnes of food and drink.
- The average digestive tract is roughly the length of a double-decker bus.
- The acids in your stomach are so strong they are similar to those used in industrial metal cleaner.

A final word

Stay Weight Wise

Maintaining a healthy weight or waist with a balanced diet and active lifestyle is important to reduce the risk of cancer. It also helps you feel great on a day to day basis, and keep you mentally as well as physically on the ball. If you are overweight, it can be useful to remember that striving for some mythical 'ideal' can be more of a hindrance than a help – big benefits can come from first stopping weight gain, then aiming for realistic and sustainable weight or waist goals.

3 Stroke – The Essentials

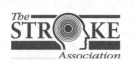

What is a stroke?

1 A stroke happens when the blood supply to the brain is suddenly disrupted. Most strokes occur when a blood clot blocks the flow of blood to the brain but some strokes can happen when a burst blood vessel floods part of the brain.

2 Sometimes a Transient Ischaemic Attack or TIA can occur. This is often called a mini stroke. The symptoms are very similar to a full-blown stroke but they do not last long – generally anything from a minute to 24 hours. TIAs can be a warning sign of a more serious problem and if you experience any of the symptoms, you should seek medical attention immediately.

3 Symptoms of a TIA are:

- Sudden numbness, weakness or paralysis on one side of the body (drooping face, arm or leg, dribbling mouth).
- Sudden difficulty speaking or understanding speech.
- Sudden blurring or loss of vision, particularly in one eye.
- Dizziness, confusion, unsteadiness and a severe headache.

What are the effects of a stroke?

4 As a stroke affects the brain – the body's central control system – the effects can be devastating. They will also vary from person to person and will depend upon which part of the brain is affected and the extent of the damage. The statistics show that in the UK one third of stroke patients will die within the first month, one third will be left with a permanent disability and one third will recover.

5 Common effects of stroke include losing the ability to swallow, becoming paralysed or weak on one side of the body (hemiplegic), suffering a range of communication difficulties, including the loss of the ability to speak, read or write and perception problems that range from having difficulty recognising and using familiar objects to complete or partial sight loss.

6 There can also be the impairment of mental processes such as memory, concentration, planning and decision making, extremes of fatigue, strong emotional reactions, including depression, mood swings, personality changes and the loss of emotional control and a loss of confidence and self-esteem. These problems are often seen in combination, reflecting the pattern and extent of an individual's brain damage. They can be temporary or permanent.

How would I recover from a stroke?

7 As the aftershock of stroke subsides, the swelling in the brain goes down and medical assessment can be made of the stroke's effects. When appropriate, a program of rehabilitation can commence, with treatments such as physiotherapy and speech and language therapy. It cannot always be determined what the recovery period after a stroke will be and people often continue to improve over many years.

8 Recovery takes place as undamaged parts of the brain learn to take over the functions of the brain cells destroyed at the time of the stroke. The rate of recovery depends very much on how well the person responds to the rehabilitation they receive.

So what's the link between obesity and stroke?

9 A stroke is totally unpredictable and there are rarely any warning signs it is about to happen. It is impossible to say why a stroke happens when it does and why some people have a stroke and others do not. The overwhelming reason is that there is a medical condition present which causes the stroke. However, the connection between lifestyle and stroke is well established.

10 As obesity is a condition that accelerates the ageing of the body, obese people commonly develop problems that would usually occur later in life such as abnormal levels of fat in the blood, high cholesterol, high blood pressure, atherosclerosis and diabetes. Thus the visible signs of obesity –

increased bulk, reduced mobility and loss of flexibility – are mirrored internally, notably in the blood and vascular system. All these conditions greatly increase the chances of a TIA or stroke occurring.

11 Studies indicate that carrying fat around the stomach can quadruple the risk of diabetes, stroke and heart disease. Women with waists over 35 inches and 40 inch waits on men are classed as high risk with regard to these conditions. Measuring your waist is a good way of assessing your future health – if you lose about 1kg in weight you lose approximately 1cm off your waist.

4 What is atherosclerosis?

1 Obesity usually reflects unhealthy dietary habits, which overload the body's systems. The bloodstream and circulation, in dealing with excessive fat and sugar intake, become prone to raised cholesterol and fat levels. So begins the process of premature atherosclerosis, or build-up of fatty plaque on the walls of arteries. This arterial debris may eventually break off and be carried round the body, causing obstruction to blood vessels in the brain and thus greatly increasing the likelihood of a Transient Ischaemic Attack (TIA) or stroke.

5 What is high blood pressure (hypertension)?

1 Your blood pressure varies throughout the day. This occurs in everyone, whether they have high blood pressure or not. It can go up if you are rushing about or stressed and go down if you are at rest. As you get older blood pressure tends to rise. High blood pressure is also more prevalent among people of African-Caribbean descent. Diabetes and other illnesses can also raise blood pressure.

2 When your blood pressure is measured, it is done when the heart beats (systolic pressure) and when the heart relaxes between beats (diastolic pressure). Both pressures are measured in millimetres of mercury, written as 'mmHg', and when blood pressure is

measured and recorded, the systolic reading is always written before the diastolic figure. Normal adult blood pressure should be less than around 140/90 mmHg.

3 A person is considered to have hypertension (high blood pressure) if they have a measurement that is consistently over 140/90 mmHg. This multiplies their risk of stroke six fold, and treatment is usually needed to bring it down.

Why is high blood pressure dangerous?

4 High blood pressure puts a strain on blood vessels all over the body, including vital arteries to the brain. The excess pressure can damage the lining of an artery, allowing blood clots to form and cause blockages. The extra strain may also cause blood vessels to burst, so that blood spills into surrounding tissues (cerebral haemorrhage). This is what causes a stroke.

How can I reduce the risk?

5 If your blood pressure is high, but below around 160/90, your doctor may initially suggest lifestyle changes which may be enough by themselves to correct it such as giving up smoking, altering your diet to lower your fat, sugar and salt intake and to increase the amount of fruit, vegetables and high fibre foods you eat, losing any excess weight, reducing

your alcohol intake, getting regular exercise and trying to reduce your stress levels.

6 If these lifestyle changes do not reduce your blood pressure to normal, there are a variety of medicines which your doctor can prescribe. These will in some cases have side effects, so that it may take time to find a workable treatment. This will have to be followed for the rest of your life.

6 Cholesterol and heart disease

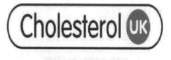

A joint initiative of H•E•A•R•T UK
and the British Cardiac Patients Association

Prepared by Angie Jefferson, Consultant Dietician

1 Cholesterol – we can't see it and we can't feel it, but we all have it and while we need some cholesterol for good health, most of us have too much which is where the problems start. The fact is that for most of us, our cholesterol levels are too high because of what we eat and how we live our lives. However the news is not all bad – we can take steps to lower our cholesterol levels and give

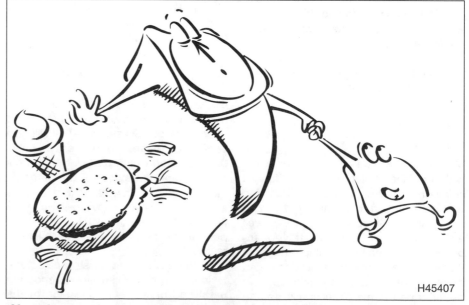

H45407

Your doctor may suggest lifestyle changes such as altering your diet to lower your fat, sugar and salt intake

ourselves a better chance of a long and healthy life with a lowered risk of developing heart disease.

The facts

Cholesterol

- Cholesterol levels are directly related to the risk of developing heart disease and strokes.
- People who are obese are not only likely to have high cholesterol, but are also likely to have poor glucose tolerance and raised blood clotting factors – greatly increasing the risk of heart disease and strokes.
- Half of all cases of heart disease are estimated to be due to having raised cholesterol levels.
- Two thirds of men and women have higher than ideal cholesterol levels.
- People with high cholesterol are more likely to get a build up of cholesterol in the arteries of the heart, brain, pelvic and abdominal arteries, causing heart attacks, strokes and contributing to impotence.
- 8 out of 10 people do not know they have raised cholesterol.
- Cholesterol levels can be lowered by dietary changes, in particular less saturated fat, using plant stanols or sterols, foods containing soya, oily fish, being more active and drug therapy.
- A proportion of people with elevated cholesterol levels will need medication.
- Losing weight reduces cholesterol, blood clotting and risk of heart disease. A 10kg weight loss is likely to result in:
    A 10% fall in total cholesterol.
    A 15% fall in LDL (bad) cholesterol.
    A 30% fall in triglyceride levels.
    An 8% increase in HDL (good) cholesterol.

Heart Disease

- Heart disease is the biggest single cause of death in the UK – the third highest rate in Western Europe behind Finland and Ireland.
- More than 65,500 men die of heart attacks each year (1 every 8 minutes).
- A British male of working age is twice as likely to die from heart disease as an Italian male.
- A Scottish man is 50% more likely to die prematurely from heart disease than a man in the south west of England.

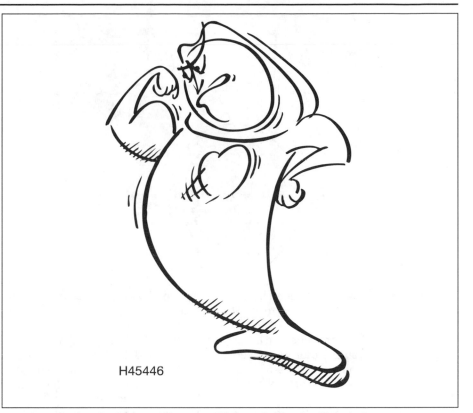

H45446

Look after your heart and keep cholesterol levels low

- A manual worker is 58% more likely to die of heart disease than a non-manual worker.
- South Asian men living in the UK (Indian, Pakistani, Bangladeshi or Sri Lankan) have a rate of heart disease 46% higher than white men. And this difference is increasing!
- Despite more people surviving heart attacks, the number of people with heart disease is increasing in the UK – 1.5 million men in the UK have had a heart attack or live with angina.
- Death rates from heart disease have fallen but increasing rates of overweight and obesity could reverse this trend.

2 Get the picture? Looking after your heart and keeping cholesterol levels low is important for all men, of all ages. The facts are hard but there is nowhere to hide – cholesterol causes heart disease which kills men (and women) – and many of these deaths are unnecessary. You may believe that it will never happen to you – but the risk is real, it could happen to you, and sooner than you think, so the choice is yours whether to do something to look after yourself and reduce your risk or take your chances that everything will be alright.

What is cholesterol?

3 Cholesterol is an off-white waxy substance – a type of fat, which is carried around in the bloodstream in particles called lipoproteins. There are two different types of cholesterol: Low Density Lipoprotein (LDL) cholesterol, often known as the 'bad' cholesterol, and High Density Lipoprotein (HDL) cholesterol, referred to as the 'good' cholesterol.

4 Around 80% of cholesterol is made by the body in the liver, using saturated fat from food as basic building blocks. LDL carries cholesterol from the liver to the tissues. HDL is able to recycle cholesterol from tissues that have too much cholesterol.

5 Cholesterol is also found in some foods, such as eggs, liver, kidneys, and prawns, but this tends to account for just 20% of the body's total. For most people, the amount of saturated fat in food is therefore far more important than the amount of cholesterol.

- Low density lipoproteins (LDL or 'bad' cholesterol), carries cholesterol around the body and is the main source for cholesterol that builds up and blocks the arteries.

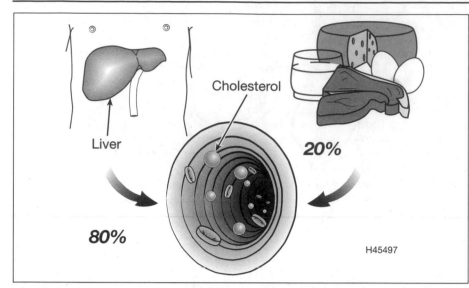

H45497

Cholesterol is mainly produced by the liver and small amounts come from the foods that we eat

- High density lipoproteins (HDL or 'good' cholesterol), returns unused cholesterol to the liver for recycling, thus helping to keep cholesterol out of the arteries.
- Triglycerides, the fats that we recognise in our food and store under the skin. Like cholesterol, triglycerides from the gut (diet) or made in the liver are also carried on the lipoprotein particles in the blood.

6 The aim is to keep LDL levels lower and HDL levels higher. The ratio of LDL to HDL is important in assessing risk of heart disease.

What does cholesterol do?

7 Cholesterol is a structural component of cells (think of the bricks and mortar in a wall) and so plays an essential role throughout the body. It is also used to manufacture vitamin D and hormones, such as testosterone and oestrogen, and to produce bile acids which help us to digest the fat that we eat. It only becomes a problem when there is too much in the wrong place – in the bloodstream.

What is a normal cholesterol level?

8 When a blood test is taken it is normal to break the test down into several parts. The first is total cholesterol, which includes measures of both the LDL and HDL cholesterol fractions, and other minor lipoproteins. From a fasting blood sample (i.e. after not eating for 8 hours), the levels of total

cholesterol, HDL and triglycerides are measured and then the level of LDL calculated from these. What is important are both the total values and the amount of the different fractions.

9 Current recommendations are for individual's levels to be:
- *Total cholesterol (TC) less than 5.0mmol/l or 190mg/dl**
- *LDL cholesterol (LDL-C) less than 3.0mmol/l or 115mg/dl*

10 Levels of HDL and triglycerides are not included in the current recommendations but a guide as to the correct levels is below:
- *HDL cholesterol (HDL-C) greater than 1.0mmol/l or 40mg/dl*
- *Triglycerides less 2.3mmol/l*

* **Note:** *In the UK lipids would usually be measured in millimoles (of cholesterol) per litre (of blood) (mmol/l), while milligrams per decilitre (mg/dl) is used in North America.*

11 These recommendations were made several years ago and are now under review. The new levels are likely to be for: total cholesterol to be less than 4.0mmol/l and LDL to be below 2.0mmol/l. If these figures are adopted then just 15% of men will have ideal cholesterol levels and just 2% a healthy LDL level.

How does cholesterol link to heart disease?

12 If we are eating a healthy diet and living a healthy life the cholesterol produced by the liver is evenly balanced with the amount that the body can deal with, picture a see-saw – with the body on one side and the liver on the other, with the see-saw evenly balanced. But for most of us the amount of cholesterol produced by the liver is far bigger than the amount the body can handle and so the see-saw is out of balance.

13 When cholesterol levels are high it begins to be deposited inside the

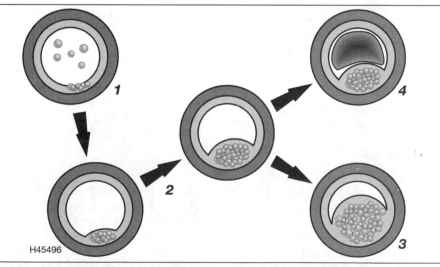

H45496

When cholesterol levels are high it begins to be deposited in the arteries

1 *Deposits begin to form in the arteries*
2 *Over time the blockages build in size*
3 *The blockage restricts blood flow and causes angina*
4 *A clot forms blocking blood flow and causing a heart attack*

arteries – similar to the build up of lime-scale inside water pipes. This process is called atherosclerosis (or hardening of the arteries). Over time the blockage builds up and reduces the amount of blood flowing through the artery. Blockage in the arteries to the heart can cause angina – an uncomfortable feeling of pressure or pain across the chest, or even reaching out to arms, neck, stomach or jaw on emotional or physical exertion, due to insufficient blood reaching the heart muscle. The fatty blockage encourages blood to clot on its surface – like a scab on a cut. If the artery blocks completely, the heart muscle starved of blood dies (the heart attack) – or when the carotid arteries to the brain are blocked, the brain cells die resulting in a stroke. Arteries in the abdomen or pelvis are also affected, potentially affecting the kidneys, sexual function or leading to leg gangrene.

What all men should know – it's not just about the heart!

Did you know that atherosclerosis can affect any of the arteries, not just those in the heart, but also those in the legs, brain, abdomen and pelvis? It is estimated that a quarter of all cases of erectile dysfunction (impotence) are caused by impaired blood flow to the penis.

So taking steps to lower cholesterol will not only look after your heart and circulation, but also increases the chances of you maintaining a healthy sex life into older age as well.

Risk factors for heart disease

14 High blood cholesterol (also referred to as hypercholesterolemia) is one of the 'major risk factors' for coronary heart disease (CHD). But cholesterol isn't the only risk factor and it's important to consider the other risk factors as well. These include:

- Smoking – the best way to cut risk is to give up. Giving up alone is hard, but your GP or Practice Nurse is specially trained to help people quit and make the best use of aids such as nicotine patches or gum.
- High blood pressure (Hypertension) makes hardening of the arteries worse and forces the heart and kidneys to

work harder than they should. High blood pressure can be lowered by weight loss, cutting back on alcohol, eating less salt and more fruit and vegetables.
- Overweight and obesity – dramatically increase the risk of developing heart disease. Losing weight is a priority to reduce cholesterol and other risk factors for heart disease.
- Physical inactivity – only one third of men are active enough for good health – i.e. undertake 30 minutes of moderate activity on at least 5 days each week. Be honest – at least 5 days a week? Most of us need to do a lot more, particularly if we need to lose weight.
- Diabetes – having diabetes greatly increases the risk of heart disease, especially if the diabetes is not well controlled.

15 Other lifestyle factors may also play a part in heart disease, including drinking too much alcohol, eating too much salt, and having raised levels of stress. And these factors don't simply add up – one factor will increase your risk, add in a second or a third and the risk multiplies. However, a raised level of cholesterol in the blood is the single greatest factor, contributing to almost half of all deaths from CHD.

How do I get my cholesterol tested?

16 There are usually no symptoms of high cholesterol so the only way to know your cholesterol level is to have a blood test. In the recent National Diet and Nutrition Survey of UK adults, more than half of all UK men had high total cholesterol, more than 80% had raised LDL cholesterol and almost half had low HDL cholesterol levels.

17 Your options for a blood cholesterol test are:

- Ask your GP or practice nurse – where you know the test will be reliable and your results can be interpreted along with any other risk factors you may have.
- Your work place – may offer heart health checks through occupational health or private clinics
- Some pharmacies will offer checks given by trained pharmacists.
- Home cholesterol kits can be purchased through pharmacies, but it is ideally recommended to obtain a test for a full lipid profile including both

your total and LDL cholesterol. Home tests, which only measure total cholesterol levels, can be inaccurate unless used extremely carefully giving you a false reassurance that your cholesterol level is normal or worrying you if your result is very high. Many patient support organisations do not advise use of home cholesterol test kits. If you do use a kit, it is worth checking your results with your pharmacist or GP to ensure you have an accurate result.

18 Ideally we should all get our cholesterol levels tested every 5 years or so, like our blood pressure, and more often if you've had a high test before. But you are especially recommended to ask your GP for a test if any of the below apply to you:

- *There is a history of heart disease or raised cholesterol in your family.*
- *You have diabetes.*
- *You have high blood pressure.*
- *You already have coronary heart disease.*
- *You smoke.*
- *You are overweight/obese.*
- *You have peripheral arterial disease (hardening of abdominal or leg arteries).*
- *You have had a previous stroke.*

19 Your GP or pharmacist should explain the results to you; let you know what the cholesterol levels mean, and if you have other risk factors.

Why do men get more heart disease than women?

20 In general women tend to have higher levels of blood pressure, total and LDL cholesterol and a greater incidence of diabetes than men. However, before the age 65, four times as many men die from heart disease as women and 3-4 times as many men will have heart attacks. This is due to several reasons. Before the menopause women are protected by the hormone oestrogen, which helps to keep HDL levels high – 3-4 times more men have low levels of "good" HDL cholesterol compared to women. In addition women tend to smoke less and are more likely to store body fat around the hips (pear shape) rather than around the abdomen (apple shape). Abdominal fat is far more damaging to health than fat stored around the hips. Once women reach the menopause and oestrogen levels fall and LDL levels rise, rates of heart disease begin to increase.

So what can I do to change my cholesterol levels?

21 Reducing cholesterol reduces risk of CHD. And the sooner you do this the better. The lower the cholesterol levels over your lifetime, the more your life long heart attack and stroke risk is reduced. Even a 10% cholesterol fall from a young age or a low level can reduce risk by more than a third.

22 A variety of things can affect cholesterol levels. These are things you can do something about:

- **Changing Diet** – eating less saturated fats, increasing intake of fibre and wholegrain foods, using plant stanols or sterols, eating foods made from soya, and more fruit, vegetables and oily fish are all important.
- **Losing Weight** – lowers LDL and triglycerides, and raises HDL cholesterol.
- **Being Active** – regular activity lowers LDL and increases HDL cholesterol.

23 There are other factors that can affect your cholesterol levels, but these are things you cannot do anything about:

- **Age and Gender** – Men have a higher risk for heart disease than women at virtually all ages. As both women and men get older, their cholesterol levels rise and risk increases. Men are more at risk of raised cholesterol than women. However women catch up – as many or more women will die of CHD.
- **Heredity** – Your genes partly determine how much cholesterol your body makes. High blood cholesterol can run in families known as familial hypercholesterolemia (FH) or familial combined hypercholesterolemia (FCH).

Drug Treatments

24 Some people with very high cholesterol levels or who have several risk factors for heart disease may also need drug therapy prescribed by their GP. The decision to embark on prescribed treatment will be taken jointly by yourself and your doctor. The most commonly prescribed drugs are statins which reduce the amount of cholesterol manufactured by the liver, and as a result lower total and LDL cholesterol quickly and effectively. For best effects these need to be taken in conjunction with the lifestyle changes outlined here.

25 Since mid-2004, statins can now also be brought over-the-counter in pharmacist stores, or from web pharmacies. If buying in store the pharmacist is likely to ask you a few questions about your health to check that these are right for you. The dosage in the statins that you can buy from the pharmacist is lower than that which would be prescribed by your GP and so these should not be used to replace prescribed statins without prior approval by your GP.

26 For most people changing diet and lifestyle will allow them to reduce their cholesterol to an acceptable level. Even if prescribed drug therapy, it is still necessary to follow a healthy diet and lifestyle, if not the effectiveness of the drugs will be reduced.

Eating for a healthy cholesterol

27 Changing your diet to lower your cholesterol need not be boring and tasteless, but may need a little more thought and planning than you are used to. Remember these are changes that you need to stick to so rather than getting all dramatic – make a number of small changes and then stick to them!

28 According to the 2002 World Health Report, published by the World Health Organisation, one third of deaths from heart disease are thought to be due to unhealthy diets, so getting it right could make a big difference.

Demystifying fat

29 Dietary fat comes in different shapes and sizes, all of which have different effects on cholesterol levels. Fat is the most concentrated source of calories in the diet – providing 9kals in every gram, which is more than alcohol (7kcal/g), protein (4kcal/g) or carbohydrates (4kcal/g). What this means is that if you eat a food that is very high in fat – e.g. butter or margarine, a small amount will add a lot of calories and fat to the diet. Every one of those tiny butter pats or tubs of margarine served in restaurants contains more than 8g of fat and over 75 calories – so just imagine what's in the large blob tucked into your jacket potato or in your plate of fish and chips. Much of the fat in our diet (70%), however, comes from invisible fats such as cakes, biscuits and fatty meat products.

30 A cholesterol lowering diet does not necessarily mean that you have to cut out all fats – it does however mean that you need to cut down on fat, especially saturated and trans fat, while using monounsaturated or polyunsaturated fats instead (see below). If you need to lose weight, keeping your intake of all fats low will make this easier.

31 You can learn a lot about the fat content of foods by checking the nutrition label on the side of the pack. This tells you the total amount of fat and, on many packs, also the amount of saturated fat in the food. Start to compare labels and choose brands with lower total and saturated fats.

32 As a general guide – if you are not overweight a maximum intake of fat is 95g per day and if you need to lose weight aim for less than this e.g. 70g fat per day. In terms of saturates a maximum of 30g saturated fat each day – although to lower cholesterol a maximum of 20g per day is a better target.

News Flash
Decreasing dietary saturates (saturated fat) can help lower blood cholesterol.

Saturated fats

33 Most people in the UK eat a diet that contains high levels of saturated fat, and this is a major reason why many of us have high cholesterol levels. It's quite simple – the body uses saturated fats to manufacture cholesterol and so limit the saturated fat and the body makes less cholesterol. Foods high in saturated fat include: animal products such as fatty cuts of meat, sausages and meat products like pies and sausage rolls; full fat dairy products; butter, ghee, lard, cream; hard cheese; cakes, pastries and biscuits; chips and savoury snacks.

Unsaturated fats – Monounsaturates and Polyunsaturates

34 Replacing saturated fats with either monounsaturates (MUFA) or polyunsaturates (PUFA) can reduce total and LDL cholesterol levels. MUFA offer some advantages over PUFA as they reduce total and LDL-cholesterol without adverse effects on HDL cholesterol or triglyceride levels.

A guide to choosing fats and oils

Saturated Limit use	Polyunsaturated OK in moderation	Monounsaturated OK in moderation
Butter	Corn oil or spreads	Hazelnut or peanut oil
Ghee – butter or palm	Soya oil or spreads	Olive oil
Coconut oil	Sunflower oil or spreads	Rapeseed oil
Lard	Walnut or sesame oil	Mustard seed oil
Palm oil	Grapeseed oil	
Suet	Safflower oil	
	Plant stanol or sterol spreads	

Fat swaps

35 Most fat, and saturated fat comes from spreads such as butter, milk, meat pies, cakes, biscuits, burgers, sausages, you may think you have to give up foods you eat and enjoy and there will be no pleasure left in eating. But it's worth looking at how a few food swaps can really make a difference in lowering the saturated fat.

Instead of	Try this	Total fat saving	Saturated Fat Saving
Butter spread on 2 slices bread	Polyunsaturated margarine	2 grams	5 grams
1 pork loin chop, grilled lean and fat	1 pork loin chop, grilled lean only	11 grams	4 grams
1 medium sausage roll (puff pastry)	Ham salad sandwich	8.5 grams	5 grams
120g portion steak and kidney pie pastry top & bottom	120g steak and kidney pie, pastry top only	8 grams	4 grams
BLT sandwich	Tuna mayonnaise sandwich – use low fat mayo	7.5 grams	3 grams
1 tablespoon ordinary mayonnaise	1 tablespoon lite mayonnaise	11.9 grams	1.8 grams
30g packet crisps	1 banana	10 grams	4 grams
1/2 pint whole milk	1/2 pint semi-skimmed milk	5 grams	4 grams
1 jam doughnut	1 slice of malt fruit loaf	10 grams	3 grams
Small (50g) bar dairy milk chocolate	50g liquorice allsorts	13 grams	7.4 grams
Quarter pounder with cheese	Quorn™ burger	21 grams	9 grams
1 takeaway large portion fries	1 takeaway regular portion fries	9 grams	2 grams
1 portion fried chips (265g)	1 portion oven chips (265g)	22 grams	4 grams
Cheese and pickle sandwich	Egg mayonnaise sandwich – use low fat mayo	10 grams	10 grams
40g portion cheddar	20g portion cheddar	7 grams	4 grams
40g portion cheddar	40g portion half fat cheddar	7 grams	5 grams
350g portion beef curry	210g lentil curry dhal made with tomatoes and vegetable oil	43.5 grams	10 grams

Fishy Business – omega 3 fatty acids and fish oils

36 The omega 3 fats found in oily types of fish are another type of polyunsaturated fat, but these ones are special. Omega 3 fats have a particular role in helping to keep the arteries supple and healthy, and make the blood less likely to clot inside blood vessels (clots cause heart attacks and strokes). Oily types of fish like herring, mackerel, sardines, salmon and fresh tuna are the best sources of omega 3s in the diet as the body is able to use these omega 3 fats directly. Try to eat these once or twice each week. If you have already had a heart attack or stroke, try to make this 2-3 times each week.

37 Non-fish sources of omega 3 fats include rapeseed oil, linseed, walnuts and seeds such as pumpkin seeds.

Trans fats

38 Like saturated fats, trans fats can raise cholesterol levels. Trans fats are found in foods that contain processed (hydrogenated) fats, including some types of biscuits, cakes, fast food, pastry, margarine and spreads. So, as part of a healthy diet, try to cut down on foods containing hydrogenated or saturated fats and replace them with unsaturated fats. You will need to check the labels on these types of foods.

Tips to cut fat

39 A quick reminder – the cholesterol in food only has a small impact on the cholesterol in the body – it is more important to concentrate on reducing total and saturated fats.

- Choosing how to cook foods well can make a big difference to your fat intake. Try to choose cooking methods such as microwaving, steaming, poaching, boiling or grilling, instead of roasting or frying and choosing lean cuts of meat and low-fat varieties of dairy products and spreads to help to reduce total fat.
- When using oils, always measure them out using a spoon rather than sloshing them into the pan – this way you will almost always use less.
- Buy a griddle pan to cook fish, chicken and lean steaks or burgers.
- Buy an oil in a spray can to use on salads.
- Cut back on cheese – enjoy a small amount of a strong cheese rather than a large serving of mild cheese.
- Have thicker bread and thinner spread.
- Always buy lean cuts of meat and cut visible fat off before cooking.

Carbohydrates

40 Although carbohydrate has no direct effect on blood cholesterol levels, increasing the amount of carbohydrate rich foods that you eat, while decreasing fat is usually encouraged; and after all is part of the message for general healthy eating. Choosing foods that are wholegrain – such as breads and breakfast cereals will help to keep your cholesterol low and help with weight control.

News Flash
The inclusion of oats as part of a diet low in saturated fat and a healthy lifestyle can help reduce blood cholesterol.

41 Oats contain a particular type of fibre called soluble fibre which makes them special when it comes to cholesterol.

Eating a diet rich in soluble fibre has been found to help reduce total and LDL cholesterol levels. And it's not just oats that contain soluble fibre, other good sources include pulses e.g. kidney beans, lentils and baked beans; oats, barley or rye; and fruits and vegetables.

Fruit and Vegetables

42 Unless you have been hiding under a rock for the past few years you will know that eating plenty of fruit and vegetables every day is vital for great health. The average guide is to eat at least 5 servings each day which is equivalent to 400g, but estimates are that between one quarter and one half of deaths from heart disease in countries like the UK are due to eating less than 600g of fruit and vegetables every day – so for the best heart health at least 7 servings each day is required as recommended in some other European countries. Any fruit and vegetables provide lots of vitamins and minerals but different colours provide different amounts of 'antioxidants' which help to look after the heart. Including a variety of different colours and types will increase the range of nutrients you are giving your body.

What is a serving?

An easy way to think of a serving is to think of the amount you can hold in your hand, but while this is easy with a bunch of grapes it is somewhat harder when it comes to frozen vegetables. Using the table will give you a start on different amounts of fruits and vegetables to choose. As often happens with guidelines there are a few exceptions and here are the ones to remember:

- *Pure fruit juice can only be counted once a day, no matter how much you drink.*
- *Potatoes are counted as starchy carbohydrate so don't fit in the fruit and vegetable group.*
- *Pulses and beans can count too but can only be counted once a day.*

Fruits	Example of average portion
Medium sized fresh fruit	1 apple, banana, pear, orange, nectarine
Small sized fresh fruit	2 plums, 2 satsumas, 3 apricots, 2 kiwi fruit, 7 strawberries, 14 cherries, 6 lychees
Large fresh fruit	Half a grapefruit, 1 slice of papaya, 1 slice of melon (2 inch slice), 1 large slice of pineapple, 2 slices of mango (2 inch slice)
Dried fruit	1 tablespoon of raisins, currants, sultanas, 1 tablespoon of mixed fruit, two figs, three prunes, one handful of banana chips
Tinned fruit (unsweetened)	Roughly the same quantity of fruit that you would eat as a fresh portion: 1 pear or peach half, 6 apricot half, 8 segments of tinned grapefruit
Juice	1 medium glass (150ml) of 100% pure fruit juice, but juice only counts as once a day, no matter how much you drink

Vegetables	
Green vegetables	2 broccoli spears, 8 cauliflower florets, 4 heaped tablespoons of kale, spring greens or green beans
Cooked vegetables	3 heaped tablespoons of cooked vegetables such as carrots, peas or sweetcorn
Salad vegetables	3 sticks of celery, 2 inch piece of cucumber, 1 medium tomato, 7 cherry tomatoes
Tinned and frozen vegetables	Roughly the same quantity as you would eat as a fresh portion: 3 heaped tablespoons of tinned or frozen carrots, peas or sweetcorn
Pulses and beans	3 heaped tablespoons of lentils, kidney, cannelloni or butter beans or chick peas (Remember that beans or pulses only count as one of your 5 a day portions.)

News Flash
The inclusion of at least 25g soya protein per day as part of a diet low in saturated fat can help reduce blood cholesterol.

43 Soya and foods made from this humble bean can lower cholesterol. Gone are the days of soya being a food for health freaks sold in health food stores. Soya products are now widely available in supermarkets and include great tasting products such as milks (try the fresh varieties from the chiller cabinet – great for making smoothies and shakes), yoghurts, desserts, custards. Soya is also used to make tofu – sold in a block for stir fries or as burgers, sausages or ready meals. Soya protein is also added to some breads. In order to eat 25g of soya protein in a day you will need to include a soya product on several occasions e.g. a soya smoothie for breakfast, a tofu burger for evening meal and toasted soya bread for an evening snack.

Plant Stanols and Sterols

44 Products containing plant stanols or sterols are designed specifically for people with raised cholesterol. Plant stanols and sterols are extracted from vegetable oils, concentrated and then added back into low fat spreads, yoghurts, bars and milk. One shot pots of yoghurt style drink containing a day's worth of plant stanols or sterols have recently arrived on the shelves, making using these everyday a little easier. Clinical trials have clearly shown that daily consumption of stanols or sterols can reduce LDL cholesterol by approximately 10-15%, and this is in addition to any reductions achieved by other dietary modifications or the cholesterol-lowering medications known as statins. They have no effect on HDL cholesterol. It is important to check the label and only use the amounts recommended. Tests have shown that using more than this will not increase the cholesterol reduction that you achieve. However they only work while you take them, so daily use is recommended for the best results.

Frequently Asked Questions

45 There are bound to be some myths or ideas about cholesterol that you pick up from the media, friends, advertising or just general reading. Check out the questions below and the evidence for or against their truth.

Does garlic reduce cholesterol?

Minimally. Some studies have suggested that garlic may reduce cholesterol levels but there is not enough quality evidence to show that it has any effect.

Does too much caffeine increase cholesterol levels?

Despite numerous studies there is little evidence to link caffeine and cholesterol levels. It is advisable to limit coffee consumption to 2 or 3 cups per day for other health reasons and enjoy a variety of drinks to keep fluid intake up, not just coffee.

Fish oil supplements – do they work the same as oily fish?

If you have already had a heart attack or any form of cardiovascular disease, then you should include large portions of oily fish 2 to 3 times per week; or it can be taken in equivalent fish oil supplements (check they contain 0.5-1.0 grams omega 3 fatty acids per day) or rapeseed oil. Both eating oily fish and taking fish oil supplements appear to reduce heart disease.

Do probiotics help prevent raised cholesterol?

Although probiotic bacteria can possibly help with gut function and immunity there is little evidence supporting a role for them in cholesterol lowering. One shot probiotic drinks look very similar to those containing plant stanols and sterols – so check carefully to avoid confusion.

Does alcohol affect cholesterol levels?

Small amounts of alcohol (1-2 units/day) may slightly boost HDL levels. However, alcohol is high in calories so can contribute to overweight which will raise cholesterol negating effects on HDL. Alcohol has a direct effect on triglycerides so if yours are raised you need to cut right back on alcohol.

Summary

46 Raised blood cholesterol is one of the most important risk factors in predicting coronary heart disease. But lowering it is quite achievable, you don't need to be a kill joy and give up all of your favourite foods. Think of it positively and take the opportunity to try all those foods you may not have tried before and that can help lower your cholesterol. See the 10 points below. However one pretty important fact to recognise is that this diet is for life, a week won't do or even a few months. To maintain healthy levels of cholesterol and help work on maintaining weight, you need to recognise this is a permanent change.

47 We all know that small changes can make a difference and following any of the points summarised here is a good start, but the more of them you are able to do, the bigger difference it will make.

- Only buy a margarine or spread that says high in monounsaturated fat (MUFA) or polyunsaturated fat (PUFA).
- Try to use olive oil for cooking and nut oils for salad.
- Get used to carrying fruit or vegetables with you or having them handy at home. Biscuits and cakes are usually more readily available and can make an easy tempting alternative.
- Ask your local food outlet where you go for meals or snacks to always have some fresh and tasty fruits and vegetables very visible.
- Do some food swapping – those pies and pastries are loaded with saturated fats and a bap, wrap, baguette or sandwich is usually a better choice if you watch the amounts of cheese and mayonnaise.
- Make up your own sandwich with thick slices of bread; choose a moist filling so you can leave out the spread or mayonnaise.
- A small change in cooking habits – measuring the unsaturated fat you use, grilling, steaming or microwaving can go quite a way to reducing saturated fat.
- What about giving some soya products a try – chilled fresh soya milk is an easy start; to drink, add to cereal or a quick smoothie. Add tofu to a stir fry or try food that uses a tofu base such as tofu sausages or burgers.
- When you think of food, think activity – try to fit in a quick walk at lunchtime, or in the evening whenever you can. Why not try an activity you haven't tried before.
- Always have breakfast – wholegrain cereal, porridge with fruit or wholegrain toast. If you don't like wholegrain try a 'half and half' variety.

References

Joint British Recommendations on prevention of coronary heart disease in practice: summary. *BMJ* 2000 Vol 320:705-708

Royal Pharmaceutical Society of Great Britain. Practice Guidance on: Cholesterol Testing. June 2003, version ii. Available at: http://www.rpsgb.org.uk/ Accessed on: 20 September 2004.

British Heart Foundation CHD heart disease statistics 2003 & 2004

Department of Health (1996) Strategy statement of Physical Activity. DH:London

Law MR, Wald NJ, Thompson SG. By how much and how quickly does reduction in serum cholesterol concentration lower risk of ischaemic heart disease? *BMJ* 1994; 308:367-73

Tang JL, Armitage JM, Lancaster t et al. Systematic review of dietary intervention to lower blood total cholesterol in free-living subjects. *BMJ* 1998; 316: 1213-20

Silagy CS, Neil HAW. Garlic as a lipid lowering agent – a meta analysis. *J Roy Coll Phys* 1994; 28:39-45

Myers MG, Basiniki A. Coffee and coronary heart disease. *Arch Intern Med* 1992; 152:176-72

Kleemola P, Jousilahki P, Peitinen Pet al. Coffee consumption and risk of coronary heart disease and death. *Arch Intern Med* 2000; 160:3393-400

Bucher, HC, Hengstler, P, Schindler, C. & Meier, G. N-3 polyunsaturated fatty acids in coronary heart disease: a meta analysis of randomised controlled trials. *Am J Med*. 2000; 112: 298-304

Further information

48 If you would like to know more, look in the Contacts section at the back of the book, or contact:
Information on different drug therapies can be had from NHS Direct.
Website: www.nhsdirect.nhs.uk
Lots of examples of fruit and vegetable portion sizes are on the 5 a day web site.
Website: www.5aday.nhs.uk

7 Weight and sleep

People who sleep less are much more likely to be overweight. For example individuals who sleep for only 2-4 hours per night are known to be almost twice as likely to be obese as those who sleep normally. Recently, researchers have found that sleep loss leads to altered levels of two hormones linked to appetite. One hormone, called ghrelin, is produced by the stomach and stimulates hunger. The other, called leptin, is produced by fat cells, and low levels of this are linked with a desire to eat. People who sleep for 5 hours or less have 15% more ghrelin and 15% less leptin than those who sleep for 8 hours. These hormonal changes may cause increased feelings of hunger, and cause overeating.

Research suggests that lack of sleep may be contributing to growing levels of obesity. The average adult now sleeps up to two hours a night less than 50 years ago because of increasing pressures on our time (work, school, family, television, computer games and the internet). Good sleep, combined with other lifestyle changes, may therefore be an important factor in fighting obesity.

Ironically, obesity can also contribute to poor sleep by causing sleep apnoea. 'Apnoea' is a medical term, which means 'not breathing'. Sleep apnoea therefore means episodes during sleep when the breathing stops, usually caused by obstruction to the airway in the throat or neck. Typically, somebody who suffers from sleep apnoea will recurrently stop breathing throughout the night, usually for periods of 15-20 seconds, up to every minute. It is usual for the sufferer to be completely unaware of this problem while asleep, although partners will be aware that they are snoring heavily and may stop breathing for brief periods. What tends to happen is that the snorer will wake momentarily, move, take a breath, and then immediately drop back to sleep with no conscious memory of waking. Obviously if this is happening dozens or hundreds of times through the night, it will severely affect sleep quality. Sufferers will wake feeling unrefreshed (often with a headache), and may feel severely sleepy during the day, even if they have had a normal quantity of sleep. This daytime sleepiness can be very dangerous, as it can cause an increased risk of accidents especially when driving. There are also long-term medical risks, with an increased danger of high blood pressure, heart disease and strokes.

Sleep apnoea affects about 1 in 20 adults, and is twice as common in men as in women. Only 1 in 40 people who have it are aware that they have it. Being overweight is the single most important risk factor: this more than doubles the risk of the problem, particularly if there is a large collar size (over 17 inches) as well. Extra fat in the neck squashes the throat from outside, particularly when the throat muscles become floppier with sleep. Other factors can also contribute to sleep apnoea, such as smoking, having large tonsils or a slightly small jaw. Pillow size is important, as individuals who sleep with two or more pillows are more likely to obstruct their airway when asleep. Alcohol also relaxes the neck muscles during sleep, and can cause or aggravate the condition.

If you think that you have sleep apnoea, then you should see your doctor. They may wish to refer you for further assessment. Specialist treatments can include CPAP (which is a type of pump that helps to blow air into the airway through a face mask while asleep), splints to help keep the jaw forward when asleep, or surgery. However the first, and perhaps the most important stage in treatment, is to lose weight (and if necessary stop smoking or reduce your alcohol consumption). Losing weight may therefore significantly help your sleep quality, and improving your sleep quality may help you to lose yet more weight.

Chapter 7
Eating disorders and men

Contents

1 Introduction

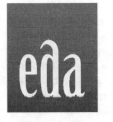

1 Food and eating play a very important part in our lives. We all vary in the foods we like, how much we need to eat, and when we like to eat. Food is essential for our health and development. It's not unusual to experiment with different eating habits, for example you may have decided to become a vegetarian or tried changing your diet to improve your health. However, some eating patterns can be damaging.

2 Problems with food can begin when it is used to cope with those times when you are bored, anxious, angry, lonely, ashamed or sad. Food becomes a problem when it is used to help you to cope with painful situations or feelings, or to relieve stress, perhaps without you even realising it. If this is how you deal with emotions and feelings, and you are unhappy about it, then you should try to talk to someone you trust. Try not to bottle things up – this is not helpful to you or other people around you, it won't make you feel any better and the problem is unlikely to go away.

3 It is unlikely that an eating disorder will result from a single cause. It is much more likely to be a combination of many factors, events, feelings or pressures which lead to you feeling unable to cope. These can include: low self-esteem, family relationships, problems with friends, the death of someone special, problems at work, college or at university, lack of confidence, sexual or emotional abuse. Many people talk about simply feeling 'too fat' or 'not good enough'. Teasing or even bullying around weight and shape have been identified as specific triggers for men.

4 Often people with eating disorders say that the eating disorder is the only way they feel they can stay in control of their life, but as time goes on it isn't really *you* who is in control – it is the eating disorder. Some people also find they are affected by an urge to harm themselves or misuse alcohol or drugs. You may find that in common with many other people you experience feelings of despair and shame. You may have a feeling of failure or lack of control because you cannot overcome these feelings about food on your own.

2 Who do eating disorders affect and when?

1 Anyone can develop an eating disorder, regardless of age, sex, cultural or racial background, usually they appear around 14 to 25, however it's not unusual for an eating disorder to appear in middle age. There also seems to be a slightly higher incidence of eating disorders amongst the gay population.

2 Many people assume that eating disorders only affect teenage women. This is not true. At least 10% of people *diagnosed* as having an eating disorder are men. However there are probably many more undiagnosed cases because there is less chance of the condition being recognised in male sufferers. Many men find it hard to ask for help especially when the doctor or counsellor does not recognise their symptoms.

3 One of the most common symptoms of eating disorders in males is an excessive concern about fitness leading to over-exercising. This can put excessive pressure upon joints and lead to muscular complaints. It may also strain heart and lungs.

4 Research has shown that your genetic make-up may have a small impact upon whether or not you develop an eating disorder. Even the attitude of other family members towards food can have an impact. A key person – a parent or relative – may unwittingly influence other family members through his or her attitude to food. In situations where there are high academic expectations, family issues or social pressures, you may focus on food and eating as a way of coping with these stresses. Traumatic events can sometimes trigger an eating disorder: bereavement, being bullied or abused, an upheaval in the family (such as divorce), long term illness or concerns over sexuality. Someone with a long-term illness or disability – such as diabetes, depression, blindness or deafness – may also experience eating problems.

5   It's important to know that everyone will not have the same symptoms. Some people will have a mix of symptoms and you do not need to have all these symptoms to have an eating disorder.

3   Anorexia Nervosa

1   'Anorexia nervosa' (often shortened to anorexia) means 'loss of appetite for nervous reasons' but this is misleading because in reality you have lost the ability to allow yourself to satisfy your appetite. You probably restrict the amount you eat and drink, sometimes to a dangerous level. You may exercise to burn off what you perceive to be excess calories. You focus on food in an attempt to cope with life, not to starve yourself to death. It is a way of demonstrating that you are in control of your body weight and shape. Ultimately, however, the disorder itself takes control and the chemical changes in the body affect the brain and distort thinking, making it almost impossible for you to make rational decisions about food. As the illness progresses, you will suffer from the exhaustion of starvation. Occasionally people die from the effects of anorexia, especially if it is untreated.

The effects of anorexia on your body

2   In adults, extreme weight loss; in children and teenagers, poor or inadequate weight gain in relation to their growth or substantial weight loss.
- *Constipation and abdominal pains.*
- *Dizzy spells and feeling faint.*
- *Bloated stomach, puffy face and ankles.*
- *Downy hair on the body; occasionally loss of hair on the head when recovering.*
- *Poor blood circulation and feeling cold.*
- *Dry, rough, or discoloured skin.*
- *Loss of interest in sex, infertility.*
- *Loss of bone mass and eventually osteoporosis (thinning bones).*

Psychological signs of anorexia

- *Intense fear of gaining weight and obsessive interest in what others are eating.*
- *Distorted perception of body shape or weight.*
- *Denial of the existence of a problem.*
- *Changes in personality and mood swings.*
- *Becoming aware of an 'inner voice' that challenges your views on eating and exercise.*

Behavioural signs in anorexia

- *Rigid or obsessional behaviour attached to eating, such as cutting food into tiny pieces.*
- *Mood swings.*
- *Restlessness and hyperactivity.*
- *Wearing big baggy clothes.*
- *Vomiting; taking laxatives.*

The long-term effects of anorexia

3   The long-term effects of anorexia on the body and mind can be alarming and severe, in particular there is a high likelihood of developing osteoporosis and there is a much higher than normal risk of developing heart disease.

4   Once you are on the path to recovery, it can take some weeks or months for the body and mind to re-adjust. Eating and drinking regularly can cause your body to become bloated temporarily. On one hand you may experience enormous hunger whilst on the other, weight gain can seem an alarming prospect. Dealing with the expectations of others around you can also be stressful. Personality and mood swings can also take a while to settle, depending on the emotional difficulties that you may be facing.

Anorexia and the family

5   Anorexia not only affects the person with the disorder – the whole family is affected. Each family is different but some common trends have been identified. People who develop anorexia have often been compliant and obedient children. They would be less likely to become angry than their brothers or sisters and would have been eager to please. They have often hidden their inner feelings and anxieties. They may fear failure and have an overwhelming desire to please and care for others. They are committed to achieving high standards set – or that they assume have been set – by parents or teachers, whereas often these high standards are self-imposed.

6   Anorexia may represent an attempt to demonstrate independence through control over food and eating. It is also very difficult for many people to understand that although food is an important issue, an eating disorder is actually all about feelings and emotions. This can lead to frustration and misunderstanding. Many carers find themselves saying in frustration something along the lines of "Why don't they just eat?"

7   Many families also find that the person with an eating disorder becomes the centre of attention which can seriously affect relationships between partners or brothers and sisters, parents, and other relatives.

4   Bulimia Nervosa

1   It was only in 1979 that bulimia nervosa was recognised by doctors as an eating disorder in its own right. The term bulimia nervosa means literally 'the nervous hunger of an ox'. The hunger, however, is really an emotional need that cannot be satisfied by food alone. After binge-eating a large quantity of food to fill the emotional or hunger gap, there is an urge to immediately get rid of the food by vomiting or taking laxatives (or both), by starving or reducing food intake, or by working off the calories with exercise in an attempt not to gain weight.

2   Bulimia is more difficult for others to notice as you tend not to lose weight so dramatically, or your weight will fluctuate. Even people close to you at home or work may not recognise the illness, so it can persist for many years undetected. People with bulimia may have demanding jobs that require them to be out-going and self-assured even when they feel inadequate inside. As with anorexia, people who develop bulimia become reliant on the control of food and eating as a way of coping with emotional difficulties in their life. You may also find you become obsessed with maintaining your weight.

3   You are most likely to develop bulimia in your late teens to early 20s. This sometimes occurs because of a belief that bulimia will help you to diet successfully where other attempts to lose weight have failed. It is also often

associated with low self-esteem or a general lack of self-confidence. You may have previously had anorexia.

The effects of bulimia on your body

- Frequent weight changes.
- Sore throat, tooth decay and bad breath caused by excessive vomiting.
- Swollen salivary glands making the face rounder.
- Poor skin condition and possible hair loss.
- Loss of interest in sex.
- Lethargy and tiredness.
- Increased risk of heart problems and problems with other internal organs.

Psychological signs of bulimia

- Uncontrollable urges to eat vast amounts of food.
- An obsession with food, or feeling 'out of control' around food.
- Distorted perception of body weight and shape.
- Emotional behaviour and mood swings.
- Anxiety and depression; low self-esteem, shame and guilt.
- Isolation – feeling helpless and lonely.

Behavioural signs in bulimia

- Bingeing and vomiting.
- Disappearing to the toilet after meals in order to vomit food eaten.
- Excessive use of laxatives, diuretics or enemas.
- Periods of fasting.
- Excessive exercise.
- Secrecy and reluctance to socialise.
- Shoplifting for food; abnormal amounts of money spent on food.
- Food disappearing unexpectedly or being secretly hoarded.

What is a binge?

4   At first you may begin to binge in an attempt to cope with emotional difficulties or to ease tension, but this can rapidly get out of control. You may find that the foods you eat are generally high in calories, carbohydrates and fat. In some circumstances, you may resort to eating things like uncooked pasta, partially defrosted frozen food or condiments, or retrieve and eat previously discarded food. As you start to feel full, feelings of guilt and shame come into your mind. It is not uncommon for people to eat two, three or even four times a normal amount of food in one go. In desperation, you may

vomit or take laxatives to purge yourself of everything you have consumed. At this point, some people describe feeling emotionally relieved and physically light-headed. This cycle can keep inner pain and unhappiness at bay – but only for a brief time.

5   The frequency of these bulimic cycles will vary from person to person. You may suffer from an episode every few months or if you are more severely ill, you may binge and purge several times a day. Some people may vomit automatically after they have eaten any food. Others will eat socially but may be bulimic in private. Many people do not regard their illness as a problem, whilst others despise and fear the vicious and uncontrollable cycle they are trapped in.

Long-term effects of bulimia

6   In a similar way to anorexia, bulimia can take over the life of the person with the disorder, making them feel trapped and desperate. Bingeing, purging and dramatic loss of fluids can cause physical problems which can usually be corrected once the body is nourished in an even and moderate way.

7   Bulimia can, in extreme cases, be fatal due to heart failure. An imbalance or dangerously low levels of the essential minerals in the body can significantly, even fatally, affect the working of vital internal organs. Other dangers of bulimia include rupture of the stomach, choking, and erosion of tooth enamel, painful swallowing and drying up of salivary glands. Laxative abuse can lead to serious bowel problems.

5   Binge Eating Disorder (BED)

1   Like bulimia, binge eating disorder has only recently been recognised as a distinct condition, it was first acknowledged as a disorder in its own right in 1992. BED shares some of the characteristics of bulimia but the essential difference is that you binge uncontrollably but do not purge. It is believed that many more people suffer from binge eating disorder than either anorexia or bulimia nervosa. Because of the amount of food eaten, many people with BED become obese, this can lead to problems with blood pressure, heart

disease and a general lack of fitness. The treatment for BED is in some ways similar to that for bulimia.

Signs of binge eating

- Eating much more rapidly than usual.
- Eating until feeling uncomfortably full.
- Eating large amounts of food when not physically hungry.
- Eating alone because of embarrassment at the quantities of food consumed.
- Feeling out of control around food.
- Feeling very self conscious eating in front of others.
- Feeling ashamed, depressed or guilty after bingeing.
- Being unable to purge yourself or compensate for the food eaten.

2   Compulsive overeating is a variation on binge eating when you will eat at times when you are not hungry. This may happen all the time, or it may come and go in cycles. Most people who are compulsive eaters are overweight, and may use their weight or appearance as a shield they can hide behind to avoid social interaction, others hide behind a happy or jolly façade to avoid confronting their problems. Sufferers often have great shame at being unable to control the compulsion to eat. Compulsive overeating is a serious condition and needs professional support to ensure long term recovery.

6   Other disorders associated with eating

1   Conditions as complex as eating disorders inevitably mean that there are variations in the typical signs described here, and not all symptoms will apply to all people. In fact many people find they have a diagnosis of an Atypical Eating Disorder or Eating Disorder Not Otherwise Specified (EDNOS). These are disorders where you have some but not all of the diagnostic signs for anorexia or bulimia. You may also be diagnosed with a 'partial syndrome' eating disorder if, for example, your bulimic episodes are very infrequent.

2   Some eating problems are much more distinct, such as 'chew and spit' behaviour, when a person chews food and spits it out, rather than swallowing – normal or even large amounts of food. Another example is regurgitation when

food is swallowed, and is then brought back up into the mouth for re-chewing. Some people eat non-foods, such as paper tissues, to fill themselves up without the calorific intake. All of these behaviours are more common than many people believe and sometimes exist alongside other eating disorder symptoms. They can often be overcome with professional help.

3 Prader Willi Syndrome is not an eating disorder as such, in the sense that it does not have its roots in emotional problems, but is a genetic disorder that results in excessive eating from early childhood. People with Prader Willi Syndrome may not achieve full height growth; they may have bad temper tantrums and often have learning difficulties, all of which require specialist healthcare treatment.

4 Orthorexia nervosa is a term coined by Dr S Bratman in his book *Health Food Junkies – Orthorexia Nervosa* to describe the outcome of compulsive dietary behaviour based on eating only certain 'health' foods. It is not a recognised medical term.

7   Related problems

1 Eating disorders rarely exist in isolation. For example, anxiety, depression or obsessive compulsive disorder can accompany an eating disorder. You may find that you have related psychological or medical issues that need to be dealt with, alongside treatment for your eating problems. In extreme cases you may find that specialists will not be able to treat the eating disorder until the other issues have been dealt with.

2 There is more information available about some of the following topics on the Eating Disorders Association website and information sheets on many of these issues are also available from EDA; see Section 11 for addresses.

Alcoholism, drug dependency and substance abuse

3 Many people with an eating disorder may find that they deal with the difficult emotional issues in their life by turning to alcohol or drugs to help boost their confidence or self-esteem. At least

partial rehabilitation may be necessary before treatment for the eating disorder can commence.

Laxative and diuretic abuse

4 Laxatives are any product designed to stimulate evacuation of the bowels – they include tablets, syrups, salts, drinks, laxatives in confectionery form, and 'natural' laxatives. Diuretics remove water from the body. Laxative or diuretic abuse is when you take laxatives or diuretics frequently over a prolonged period of time or take more than the recommended dose on any one occasion.

5 Neither laxative or diuretic abuse will achieve anything other than very temporary and short term apparent weight loss. Laxatives will not reduce the amount of calories you absorb. Diuretic abuse does reduce the amount of water in the body and hence weight, however water is vital for the appropriate functioning of all the body's systems and diuretic abuse can lead to fatal complications. There are numerous and long-term medical side effects of laxative abuse that can lead to serious health problems and even fatalities.

6 So called 'slimming drugs' can also have serious side effects and should only ever be taken under medical supervision, and never to lose weight inappropriately.

Tooth Decay

7 If you have anorexia nervosa or bulimia nervosa, you may experience some problems with your teeth. You may have symptoms such as sensitive teeth, toothache, or perhaps your teeth have changed colour. Most of these problems are due to acid erosion of the surface of the teeth. This acid can come from two sources: acidic foods or drinks, and stomach acid as a result of vomiting.

8 Stomach acid washing over the teeth dissolves the enamel layer of the tooth. This may lead to the pulp and nerve endings becoming exposed and the teeth may then have to be crowned or coated. Unfortunately much of the repair work undertaken to preserve the teeth of a person with an eating disorder will be ineffective unless they stop using self-induced vomiting as a method of weight control.

9 Constant drinking or sipping low calorie 'fizzy' drinks, 'sport/energy'

drinks or fruit based drinks can also have similar effects because of the acid they contain.

10 It is important not to brush teeth after vomiting as this can make the problem worse. Using a fluoride mouthwash and then waiting several hours before brushing or eating acidic foods will reduce, but not prevent problems.

Osteoporosis

11 About one in ten men will suffer from osteoporosis or 'thinning bones' during their lifetime. However if you suffer from anorexia, and occasionally bulimia, you have a much higher risk of developing osteoporosis. It is hard to predict the onset of the problem in males because hormonal changes can be difficult to spot.

Self harm

12 Self-injury (for instance: cutting, burning or overdosing), is not an attempt at suicide or a sign of madness. It may be a form of self punishment or another means of coping with emotional problems. Self harm is quite literally harming yourself, however some people find that there is great prejudice and concern that they may harm others. Self harm is also very hard for the people who care about you to understand and is likely to cause them great distress.

8   I'm worried about telling someone about my eating disorder

1 Talking to someone you trust is an important part of recovering from an eating disorder. Covering up the symptoms, disguising the amount you eat and the way you feel, can become such a habit that talking openly about the issues in your life can seem almost impossible. Many people make excuses such as "now is not the time" or "there is no one I can trust" or "they may tell my partner or my parents".

2 It is extremely difficult to recover from an eating disorder without help from other people. Often partners and parents are grateful when they finally understand why you have been behaving so strangely. Ironically, the person with the problem often mistakenly believes their problems have been completely undetected. The secrecy and denial of eating disorders can make it difficult for you to acknowledge your problem when someone who cares talks to you about it. This creates a barrier which only you can bring down, a task that may seem an impossible challenge.

3 The 'inner voice' which many people experience can make decisions about making a move towards recovery very difficult. Often your fear of gaining weight is very frightening indeed. It also affects the way you feel other people will react, and you may think their reaction will always be negative or lacking in understanding. This is the disorder distorting your thinking process, but it can be very hard to realise this. In order to recover you will have to be ready to challenge this negative thinking, and really want to move towards recovery before you will be able to respond to people who can help you.

9 Where to turn for help

1 You can find information about eating disorders on the internet, or there are many books on the subject. However you may prefer to talk to someone about your particular circumstances on a confidential helpline.

2 Confidential helplines such as those run by EDA are there to offer a listening ear. They can help you to seek out local services including self help groups where people support each other or individual self help support by phone, mail or e-mail. Helplines can offer more information about specific issues which may concern you. If you are worried about talking to your General Practitioner (GP), they can suggest some strategies which may be helpful. The EDA helpline service is there to support anyone who is concerned about themselves or someone they care about.

3 If you are living away from home or are at college or university there may be additional support available through the student union as well as the health centre or student counselling service. If you are unsure, NHS Direct can help you to find a local GP.

4 If you would prefer faith based support there are organisations that offer this. It is possible that your cultural background or faith makes seeking secular help difficult, in which case a confidential helpline can still offer support and information.

10 Seeking treatment

1 Recovery is not easy but it is certainly achievable. Remember – you *can* get better. Recovery is always possible even after many years of illness.

2 Eating disorders are complex illnesses where both the disturbed eating pattern as well as the psychological aspects have to be considered together. Restoring a regular eating pattern and a balanced diet will allow your body to return to health and give you the strength you will need to fight the disorder. Helping you to come to terms with the underlying emotional issues will enable you to cope with difficulties in a way that is not harmful to your health.

3 Before you can get better though, YOU have to want to make a change in your life. No one else can do it for you. Family, friends and professional health workers can only help by supporting, caring and providing you with the necessary guidance to lead you down the road to recovery. People with eating disorders often have mixed feelings about 'giving up' their illness. This is because their eating habits have become established as a way of coping with their emotional difficulties.

4 For most people the first step will be to talk to your General Practitioner (GP), or if you feel uncomfortable talking to your GP perhaps you could talk to a practice nurse.

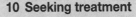

H44851

Many people with eating disorders find it difficult to talk about

5 The GP offers the easiest route to diagnosis and further treatment options through the NHS. Depending on the severity of your disorder, you may be offered a course of counselling, dietary counselling or advice, or referral to a specialist for further assessment. This may in turn lead to an offer of day-patient or outpatient treatment or, where the disorder is more serious, inpatient treatment. You may also need treatment for any medical condition which has resulted from your eating disorder, or is associated with it.

6 If you are over 16 your GP should respect your wishes if you do not want them to talk to your parents or your partner. You should talk to the GP about why you do not want them to be involved because in most cases parents or partners can be very helpful and supportive. If you are between 16 and 18 the doctor may discuss your condition with your parents if it is thought that your life is in any danger because of your eating disorder. If you are worried about who your GP might talk to or what might be said, discuss the matter first and explain your anxiety.

7 You may be so concerned about discussing your eating disorder with your GP that the words just won't come out when you are sitting in the surgery. If you are worried about being able to discuss things with the doctor, consider writing down the things that are worrying you and any questions you would like to ask. Perhaps you could take a friend or family member with you. If you feel unhappy going to a GP who may be a family friend or of the opposite sex, ask if there is another doctor in the practice you could see. If your concern is more serious you could consider moving to a new GP. NHS Direct can offer advice on moving to a new practice.

8 There are a variety of ways in which you can be treated. You may be offered a combination of different forms of therapy. If you are at a very low weight it may be essential to gain some weight before you begin therapy. You will probably be offered some form of 'talking therapy' such as: counselling, psychotherapy, cognitive analytic therapy, cognitive behaviour therapy, group therapy, family therapy. The therapy you are offered should be based on discussions between you and the

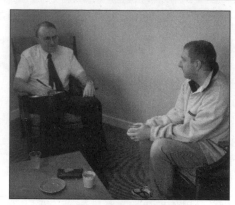
You will probably be offered counselling

healthcare professionals. If you are an in-patient or a day patient you might also be offered drama or art therapy as well as relaxation and body acceptance therapy including massage, aromatherapy or reflexology.

9 In some instances medication can help in the treatment of bulimia, or to deal with associated depression or other problems.

10 The National Institute for Clinical Excellence (NICE) guidelines for the treatment of eating disorders are the basis for most treatment in England and Wales, you can access further information on the NICE website or on the links page of the EDA website; see Section 11 for contact details. As well as the treatment guidelines NICE also publish information for patients and their carers. At the moment there are no equivalent guidelines for treatment in Northern Ireland or Scotland. EDA has a free leaflet about treatment.

11 The type of professional support you will be offered will depend upon your own particular disorder, the availability of services in your area or the arrangements that your Primary Care Trust (PCT) have made to purchase 'Out of Area Treatment Services' (OATS) from other health authorities.

Compulsory Admission

12 When you lose a great deal of weight the effects of starvation on your brain can affect your ability to think clearly. This can make any rational decisions about your own treatment or circumstances very difficult. In extreme circumstances, when all other alternatives have failed and your life or health are 'at risk', you may be fed or

treated against your will under a 'section' of the Mental Health Act. In a survey of people who had been fed or treated against their wishes, half said that, looking back, they thought it had been 'a positive thing'.

Self-help

13 Self-help may be useful as the first phase of treatment or alongside other treatments. There are many different styles of self-help publications and you need to find the right one for you.

14 Self-help groups can be a useful adjunct to treatment but, with a very few exceptions, they are not an alternative to professional treatment. However they can help sufferers and families understand they are not alone with the illness and offer valuable support and practical advice.

15 Effective treatment often involves working with families, carers and friends. The impact on the family of someone with an eating disorder can be enormous; families may also need support for themselves, and advice on what will help and what may hinder an individual's recovery, EDA helplines and support services are also there to help.

Recovering

16 Recovery can be a long haul – it is not uncommon for recovery to take five or six years, and to experience setbacks before achieving a full recovery. Nevertheless many people do recover completely.

17 If you have been an out-patient or in-patient you may find that the hardest times are just after discharge from hospital and you will certainly benefit from additional support from a counsellor, self-help group or contact at this time.

18 You may feel that your family will provide the support you need, or possibly that being apart from them would be more beneficial. In either case discuss it with them so that they understand how you feel. Support will be particularly important if you live on your own.

19 Your GP can offer some support and may be able to suggest other sources of help in your area. EDA Helplines have details of Self-help Groups and contacts all over the UK.

11 Additional help

Further information

1   If you would like to know more, look in the Contacts section at the back of the book, or contact:

Eating Disorders Association
103 Prince of Wales Road
Norwich
NR1 1DW
Tel: 0845 634 1414
Weekdays 8:30am to 8:30pm,
Saturdays 1:00pm to 4:30pm
e-mail: helpmail@edauk.com
Minicom: 01603 753 322
Weekdays 8:30am to 8:30pm
Admin: 0870 770 3256
Fax: 01603 664 915
Admin e-mail: info@edauk.com
Website www.edauk.com

Eating Disorders Association Youthline
Tel: 0845 634 7650 (Up to 18 years of age)
Weekdays, 4.00 pm to 6.30 pm,
Saturdays 1:00pm to 4:30pm
e-mail: talkback@edauk.com
txt: 07977 493 345

National Institute for Clinical Excellence (NICE)
Website: www.nice.org.uk

NHS Direct
Tel: 0845 46 47
Website: www.nhsdirect.nhs.uk

12 Eating Disorder Myths and Mythconceptions

Only middle class teenage white girls get eating disorders

Anyone can develop an eating disorder at any age, of any background, ethnic roots, gender or financial status. Eating disorders are not about who we are, they are about blocking out painful feelings and emotions and of gaining some sort of control in your life when you feel you may have lost it.

You're a bloke, men can't get eating disorders

Blokes **do** develop eating disorders, research suggests that between 10% and 20% of sufferers are male, this might be more about the fact that men visit their doctor less. It is possible the figures are actually higher.

It's just a phase

Eating disorders flourish if they are ignored and they get worse very quickly. There is strong evidence that the sooner you seek treatment the easier it is to recover. It is extremely rare for an eating disorder to just 'go away'.

I can cope by myself!

You will need support, because eating disorders are so strong, it always needs professional or guided help to beat them.

But you love cooking – you can't have a problem with food!

People with eating disorders often love cooking for others because it proves the strength of their self-control, they rarely eat any of the ingredients they prepare and it provides a good excuse for not eating with the rest of the family if the cook can pretend 'I've been snacking while I have been cooking'.

Eating Disorders are caused because no-one eats as a family any more

Again, eating disorders are more about dealing with difficult feelings and emotions as apposed to how you eat your meals. Food is not so much the issue, but the control mechanism. Even people who have been raised in families who eat together every night at the dinner table can develop eating disorders.

I'm not thin enough to be an anorexic

Don't wait until you or someone you care about is too dangerously ill to ask for help. When you have anorexia the disorder is still telling you you're not hin enough even when you don't have the strength to stand up after sitting down.

But I feel better than I ever have in my life, I feel FINE!

So that's F**ked up, Insecure, Neurotic and Emotional. Actually one of the effects of not eating enough is a 'starvation high'. You might feel full of energy in the short term, but this will soon disappear as you begin to suffer muscle wastage, shortness of breath and osteoporosis (thinning bones). For men impotence and erectile dysfunction are also likely if you do not seek treatment.

I'm intolerant to dairy products

I can't eat carbohydrates

I'm a vegan

Is that really true? People sometimes use food fads to justify both their weight loss, and inability to eat many of the things offered to them.

I can't be a real bulimic, I don't vomit, I only use laxatives and diuretics

Any form of purging means there is a problem. In fact it can be more dangerous to use laxatives and diuretics as these prevent you absorbing vitamins and minerals that you need to stay healthy. In particular you risk serious heart disease if you do not get enough potassium.

I'm not a proper anorexic, I just exercise more than the others. The thinner I am, the better I run

In the short term this may be true but as you deplete your body's reserves you will find that you hit 'the wall' sooner and sooner. You will also expose yourself to other issues that will affect your fitness such as osteoporosis and heart disease.

I don't have an eating disorder, I just binge

The most common eating disorder is Binge Eating Disorder (BED) and binging will lead to significant weight gain and may lead to other problems including depression, high blood pressure and overall loss of fitness.

We didn't have eating disorders 50 years ago, things were different then

Actually research suggest that eating disorders have always been with us in one form or another from the time we lived in caves, nevertheless just 30 years ago there was not as much awareness, consequently people were often afraid to ask for help so they suffered alone and in silence.

Glossary

Body Mass Index (BMI)

BMI or Body Mass Index can be a useful guide to both risk and recovery in adults but is very much less helpful as an indicator in children. BMI is calculated by taking your weight (in kilos) and dividing it by your height (in metres) squared (see Chapter 5).

Counselling

Counsellors can help you to see the underlying emotional difficulties causing your unhappiness and eating distress, They will help you to work out why you are using this way of coping, and to discover new ways of coping. Counsellors should be properly qualified and receive regular supervision and training.

Cognitive Therapy/ Cognitive-Behavioural Therapy

With the help of your therapist, you try to identify and change those patterns of thinking, mood and behaviour that are unhelpful because they support the eating disorder.

Dietician/Nutritionist

Someone who has studied the scientific effects of food and nutrition on the body and is able to give advice on issues relating to food and eating habits.

Psychiatrist

Someone who has initial training in general medicine as a doctor and has then specialised in the diagnosis, treatment and the prevention of mental, emotional and behavioural disorders. Psychiatrists are qualified to prescribe medication.

Psychologist

A psychologist will have a degree and further clinical training is concerned with all aspects of behaviour and the thoughts, feelings and motivation underlying such behaviour.

Psychotherapist

There are different types of psychotherapists, but all should have had specialist training to work with people to help them to resolve their difficulties. They will listen to you and use questioning techniques to try to understand your emotional issues. The exact kind of therapy will vary, but it will give you time to talk about feelings and eating problems. Whether or not it includes the whole family depends on your wishes, your family or carers and the professionals involved.

Chapter 8
Like father, like son?

Contents

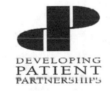

| 1 | **Regional Statistics** |

DEVELOPING
PATIENT
PARTNERSHIPS

Regional breakdown of key press release statistics from 'Get Sussed, Get Healthy Family Challenge Campaign' (DPP: Developing Patient Partnerships).

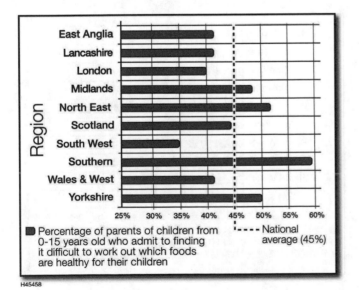

Percentage of parents of children from 0-15 years old who admit to finding it difficult to work out which foods are healthy for their children
- - - National average (45%)

H45458

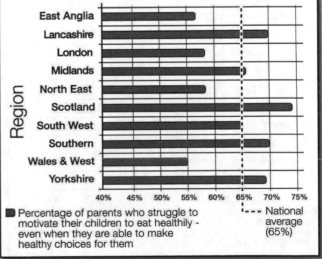

Percentage of parents who struggle to motivate their children to eat healthily - even when they are able to make healthy choices for them
- - - National average (65%)

H45459

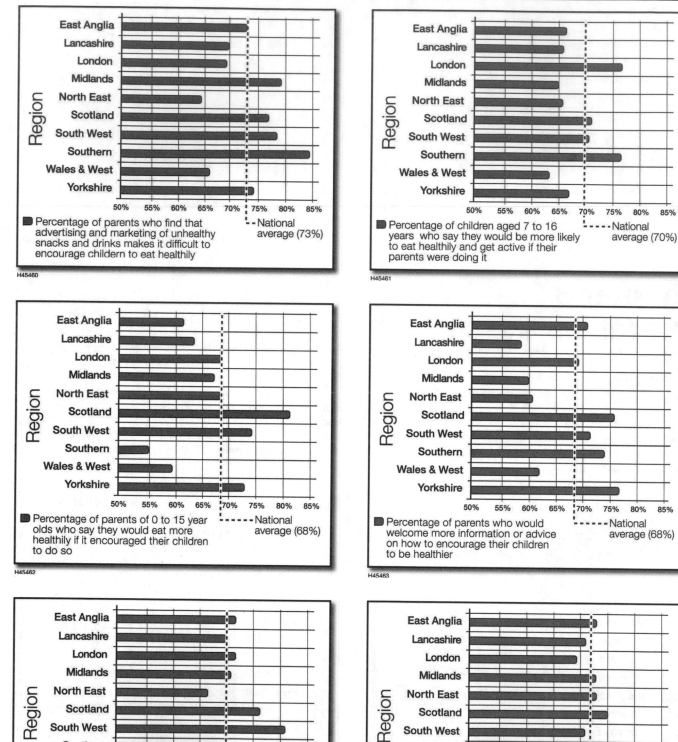

H45460

Percentage of parents who find that advertising and marketing of unhealthy snacks and drinks makes it difficult to encourage childern to eat healthily — National average (73%)

H45461

Percentage of children aged 7 to 16 years who say they would be more likely to eat healthily and get active if their parents were doing it — National average (70%)

H45462

Percentage of parents of 0 to 15 year olds who say they would eat more healthily if it encouraged their children to do so — National average (68%)

H45463

Percentage of parents who would welcome more information or advice on how to encourage their children to be healthier — National average (68%)

H45464

Percentage of parents who say that more positive messages in the media would make it easier to encourage children to be healthier — National average (75%)

H45465

Percentage who believe that schools should play a big role in teaching children how to be healthy — National average (87%)

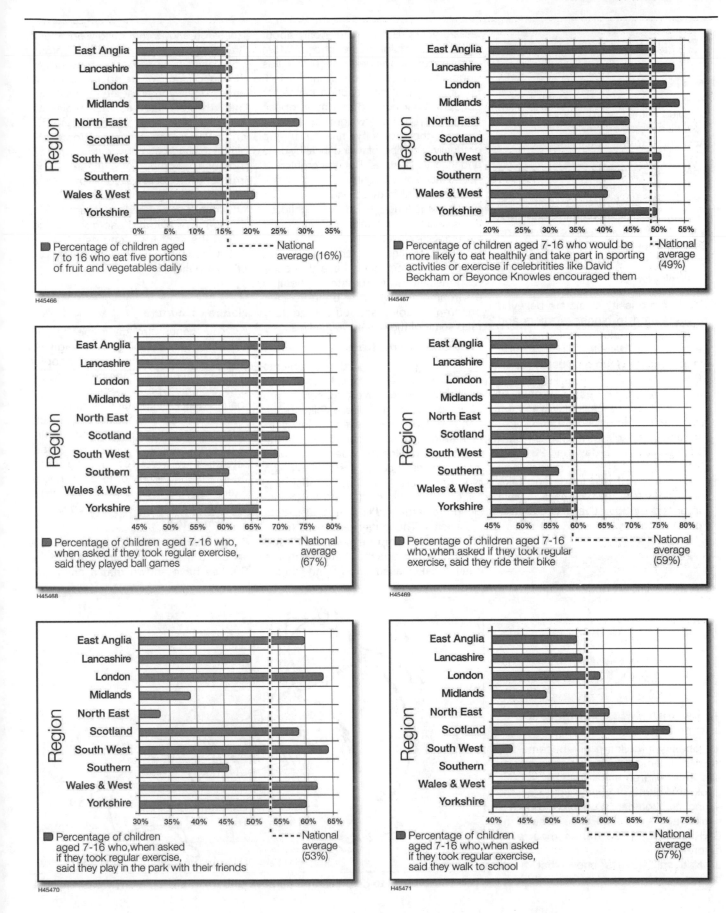

H45466
Percentage of children aged 7 to 16 who eat five portions of fruit and vegetables daily
National average (16%)

H45467
Percentage of children aged 7-16 who would be more likely to eat healthily and take part in sporting activities or exercise if celebrities like David Beckham or Beyonce Knowles encouraged them
National average (49%)

H45468
Percentage of children aged 7-16 who, when asked if they took regular exercise, said they played ball games
National average (67%)

H45469
Percentage of children aged 7-16 who, when asked if they took regular exercise, said they ride their bike
National average (59%)

H45470
Percentage of children aged 7-16 who, when asked if they took regular exercise, said they play in the park with their friends
National average (53%)

H45471
Percentage of children aged 7-16 who, when asked if they took regular exercise, said they walk to school
National average (57%)

2 Obesity Background

- The number of obese children has doubled in the last 10 years – 10% are now classed as obese.
- According to the 2001 Health Survey for England 15% of 15 year olds are obese (All Party Parliamentary Group on Obesity report 2003).
- These children are at risk from developing life-threatening conditions such as diabetes, heart disease and cancer. They also have increased risk of foot, knee and asthmatic problems – in addition, childhood obesity carries psychological consequences.
- Childhood obesity levels are believed to be related to higher fat diets and high sugar intake coupled with a sedentary lifestyle (All Party Parliamentary Group on Obesity report 2003).
- UK children drink nearly 10 cans of fizzy drink per week, eat fewer than half the recommended 5 portions of fruit and vegetables and typically burn 700 less calories a day than 20 years ago.
- Portion sizes of fast foods and take away foods over the past decade have increased by 30% (National Obesity Forum website).

3 Keeping it in the family

ASSOCIATION FOR THE STUDY OF OBESITY

The world is getting bigger – and so are our children!

1 Obesity in children has become the issue of the moment because we can all see that children have changed shape. Look at a photo of your child's class at school and compare it with your own at a similar age – the difference is striking. Children today are fatter than ever before.

2 National surveys show that frank clinical obesity in children has trebled in last 20 years. But mercifully only about 1 in 20 of children are obese. More worrying is that overweight in children has doubled and now affects around 1 in 6 children. If that isn't enough cause for concern, bear in mind that most obese adults weren't overweight children – instead their obesity has crept up gradually, a symbol of their unhealthy diets and inactive lifestyles. But, the problem is not so much overweight itself – it's the tide of ill-health that follows along too.

3 The challenge is to help children achieve and maintain a healthy weight for life. Since weight problems tend to run in families, parents who are overweight themselves have particular responsibilities to create a healthy environment in which to bring up their children. In doing so, you can actually reap some of the benefit yourselves.

Why obesity matters

4 The psychological problems associated with childhood obesity are probably the most overt consequences of being overweight. Obese children can become depressed, develop a low self-esteem and lack self-confidence. In the short-term, childhood obesity can also lead to medical conditions such as high blood pressure, poor insulin sensitivity, raised blood lipids (eg, cholesterol), sleep problems and in some cases, type II diabetes. The longer-term risks relate to the relationship between childhood obesity, adult obesity, habits and the health risks associated with these.

Research shows that childhood obesity 'tracks' into adulthood, in other words, if your child is obese now, they have a strong chance of being obese as an adult. Obesity in adult life may increase their risk of diabetes, heart disease, infertility, respiratory and joint disorders and even some cancers. Worse still, simply having been obese as a child can increase some of these risks, irrespective of whether you slim down as adults. Lifestyle habits also 'track' into adulthood; you know how tough it is to change your diet at 30 so get your kids off on the right track and help them to make positive changes now that will stick with them for life.

How did we get this big?

Nature vs. nurture

5 Your genes strongly influence your chances of becoming overweight or obese. Studies have shown that adopted children often take on the body shape of their biological parents, suggesting that 'nature' has an important influence. That said, becoming obese, ultimately, results from eating too much, not being sufficiently active, or both. The genetic effects may work by making some people feel hungrier, or less inclined to exercise, than friends who don't share their genetic predisposition to obesity.

Too much telly

6 Television watching has been directly linked to the risk of childhood obesity. Studies have shown that a child who

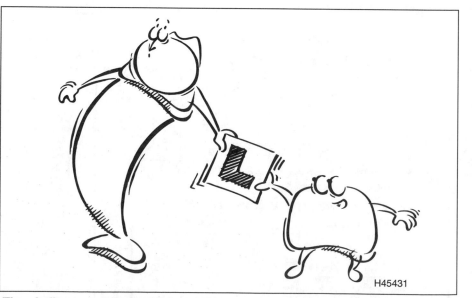

The challenge is to help children achieve and maintain a healthy weight for life

spends more than 5 hours a day watching television is 8 times more likely to become obese, compared to a child who watches fewer than 2 hours daily. The problem is made worse by poor eating habits – snacking on biscuits, crisps, etc – whilst watching telly.

You are what you eat

7 In the last 20 years we have seen portion sizes rise markedly. The problem has been worsened by 'super-sized' portions offered at favourable prices, adding financial incentives to 'Go Large'. Research has shown that people eating bigger portions are more likely to consume more calories (in part, because they do not want to waste food) but are no more likely to feel fuller for longer than someone who has eaten smaller portions of the same foods.

Couch potatoes

8 A shift towards sedentary activities – endless hours spent in front of the PC, Playstation or telly instead of being out in the park with friends, being driven to school, etc – has contributed to the rise in childhood obesity. Declines in activity have been especially marked among teenagers.

A big fat lie

9 Studies have shown that the amount of fat in your diet determines how many calories you tend to eat. Contrary to what you might think, fat-rich foods don't fill you up in the same way as calories from protein or carbohydrates, so you may be more likely to overeat.

A sweet tooth

10 Children eat more sugary foods than adults do. Children are more likely to drink sweetened, fizzy drinks, flavoured shakes or juices, snack on sweets, biscuits and cakes and have mousses, yogurts and other puddings sometimes several times a day. The biggest contributors to sugar intake in children are sweetened soft drinks. These drinks put children at an increased risk of obesity because they can be consumed in large amounts without suppressing appetite. Don't forget that these all add to their calorie intakes.

Big Daddy

11 Children born to obese or overweight parents are more at risk of weight gain than those born to parents of a healthy weight. A child with one obese parent is 20-40% more at risk of becoming obese.

This figure jumps to 80% if both parents are obese – that means that 3 out of 4 children with two obese parents are at risk of becoming obese themselves! However it's not all doom and gloom. On the positive side, any changes that you make towards lowering your own weight will benefit your kids too.

Safety fears

12 Fears about our children's safety have limited the opportunities for kids to get out and about and stay active. Adolescents are more likely to have a television and a PC rather than hang out with their friends in the park, or the street. As a result, children are now far less active they ever used to be. Just think about your own childhood and recall the things you used to get up to – playing kiss-chase or hopscotch, walking to your Gran's house or to school, biking to the shops to get something for mum, playing ball in the street, doing a paper round or washing cars in your street – and compare it to the lifestyle of your children today. Children are not inherently lazy – it's a trend that we've all nurtured. Personal safety is important but check that you are not being over-cautious.

Clinical Obesity Issues

Do my kids have fat genes?

13 Recent research has shown that a small proportion of all cases of obesity in children may be directly caused by specific genes. These genes are responsible for the body's appetite control system. Abnormalities in these genes result a voracious appetite and make it all but impossible to prevent children developing obesity. In general, children may be suspected of one of these disorders if they develop severe obesity from a very early age. If, before the age of 2 years, your child's weight exceeds most of the lines on the growth charts, if they are continuing to increase and they have a large appetite, your doctor may refer your child to a specialist centre for detailed genetic testing. Sometimes more than one member of the extended family will have had severe weight problems from an early age too.

What are the medical causes of obesity?

14 A few clinical conditions are strongly

associated with obesity. This includes syndromes such as Down's syndromes (Trisomy 21), Prader-Willi or Bardet-Biedl. You should discuss your child's weight with your hospital consultant and seek practical advice and support from dieticians and nurses involved in your child's care.

15 Some diseases or drug treatments for other conditions may be associated with sudden weight changes. This is not always fat and may often be fluid accumulation. It most cases weight may settle when the disease resolves or when treatment is completed. A small number of obese children may have a hormonal condition associated with obesity. This is usually identified and treated at an early stage. If you are worried speak to the doctor.

My child is the fattest in the class – are they obese?

16 Defining obesity in children is a difficult issue. Children naturally change shape as they grow and develop. At certain stages of life they will tend to put on more fat and at others they lose it. Differences between children in the same peer-group may just relate to their growth patterns or timing of puberty. Nonethless if you are concerned about your child's weight you should make some sequential measures of weight and height, calculate their body mass index (BMI) and plot them on growth charts available from the Child Growth Foundation. Note that the BMI calculations in Chapter 5 do not apply to growing children.

17 As a rough guide, if your child is above the 98th BMI centile you should discuss the problem with your GP. Any child falling between above the 85th and 98th BMI centile may be at risk. Look carefully at your family lifestyle, read the tips below with practical advice to help the whole family eat well and become more active. Continue to monitor their BMI once a month for the next 3 months. If they are crossing the lines on the chart in an upward direction, speak to your GP.

How quickly should my child lose weight?

18 Most children do not need to lose weight. Even if they are overweight or obese, many children will gradually grow into their size, providing they stop gaining any more weight now. With specialist advice from a health professional, children with a serious weight problem, especially after puberty, may be encouraged to lose weight gradually, at the rate of about 1-2 lbs per week.

What treatments exist for obese children?

19 Treating obesity in children is based around the same principles as adults. Changes in diet are the foundation for long-term success. The emphasis is on eating less fat and sugar and more vegetables and fruit. Learning to choose appropriate portions of food is also critical. Obese children may find it hard to exercise because of physical difficulties or worries about teasing. Children who have been overweight from an early age, may need to learn some core skills such as throwing or kicking a ball as they lose weight in order to help them start exercising.

20 Research in the USA suggests that group treatment programmes, especially those involving the whole family are the most successful in changing diet and lifestyle. Gradually more clinics specialising in treatment obesity in children are being established in the UK, but are not yet available in all parts of the country. There may also be community groups and some fitness clubs or commercial weight-loss groups may consider taking on older teenagers. Your GP or community paediatrician may be able to point you in the right direction.

21 In the UK drug treatments for obesity are not licensed for use in children. Surgery is a very last option and would rarely be considered until children have finished growing.

Further information

22 If you would like to know more, look in the Contacts section at the back of the book, or contact:

Child Growth Foundation
Website: childgrowthfoundation.org

---

4 Taking action: Helping them to help you to help them!

---

1 One of the most effective ways of losing weight and, more importantly, keeping those pounds off, is by making lifestyle changes that involve the whole family. Studies have shown that both children and adults are more likely to stay slim if they have the support of others around them, especially their family.

2 Changing eating habits and lifestyles during adolescence can be tough. It's much easier to teach your kids about the components of a healthy lifestyle before they reach their teens. If you do, the good habits are much more likely to stay with them for life and will give them with the basic tools needed to eat and exercise for long-term health. Even so, it is never too late to do something about their weight. Encourage them to adopt the action points listed below and they'll be off to a good start.

3 By following some very simple steps, you can help the whole family cut down on excess calories, learn to enjoy food and take on a new and healthy lifestyle together. As a general rule we all need to eat less saturated fat, less sugar, less salt, and more fruit and vegetables.

Diet

Size isn't everything

4 You don't need to super-size and neither do your kids. One king-sized chocolate bar provides around 20% of a 9-year old's daily energy needs. Choose a fun-sized bar instead – it's still a treat but at a smaller cost – just 5% of the day's calories.

Ready, Steady, Cook!

5 Children are more likely to enjoy their food, and try new things, if they get involved in helping to prepare it. If they reject a food the first time they try it, don't give up, tastes change fast and the more they see you having it, the greater their chances of wanting to try and like it.

Like father, like son

6 Set an example; a child is much more likely to eat healthy foods if they see other family members regularly enjoying them.

Get the breakfast habit

7 It's a fact that breakfast eaters tend to be slimmer than breakfast skippers. Eating breakfast might not turn little Jonny into Einstein, but kids who eat breakfast can concentrate for longer and perform better in short-term memory tests.

Eat meals at the table not in front of the telly

8 Show your kids that you enjoy and appreciate food, rather than treating it as a pit-stop.

Snack Attack

9 There are plenty of healthy snacks to fill everyone up between meals. Try

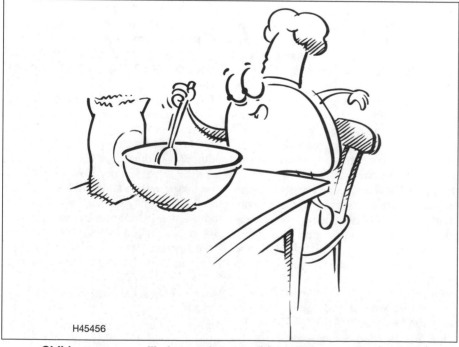

H45456

Children are more likely to enjoy new things if they are involved in preparing it

unsalted popcorn, a slice of toast, fruit or cut up pieces of vegetables, with or without home-made dips such as salsa, guacamole, hummus or natural yogurt with garlic and herbs. Fruit smoothies made with low-fat milk or yogurt can also be a great way of getting lots of vitamins and minerals whilst filling you up too.

Check out the lunch box

10 A survey by the Food Standards Agency revealed that packed lunches were providing children with more than double the recommended lunchtime intake of saturated fat and sugar, and up to half their daily salt intake. Almost half those surveyed were not getting any fresh fruit or vegetables. Crisps, biscuits and chocolate bars were common to 75% of school lunchboxes and sugary drinks found in three-quarters of cases.

11 As a general rule, try to include the following foods in their lunchbox everyday:

- *One portion of fruit and veg.*
- *One portion of low-fat milk, yogurt or cheese.*
- *One portion of meat, fish or alternatives, eg, soya, tofu, beans, etc.*
- *One portion of a starchy food, eg, bread, pasta, rice.*

Take 5

12 Everyone should be aiming to have 5 portions of fruit and vegetables each day. This could be a glass of fresh unsweetened juice, a small salad, or a banana. You can each count a portion as the size of a handful. Keep a record and see who wins at the end of week.

Watch your drink

13 Talk of a drink may turn your thoughts to alcohol, but what are your children drinking? Keeping children well-hydrated is important, but remember that colas, lemonades, squashes and even some juices can add to your calorie intake although provide few other nutrients, so try to limit these. The diet versions of some drinks are low in calories but may be bad for teeth. Wherever possible, encourage children to drink water. Skimmed or semi-skimmed milk is also a good alternative as it contains lots of essential nutrients but it also provides some calories so don't go mad! As a guide, everyone should be aiming to have 8 glasses of fluid each day.

Find new ways to reward good behaviour

14 Keep treats as occasional indulgences, not a daily bargaining tool!

Don't force your child to finish their plate if they say they are full (and don't let them have a pudding either!)

Physical Activity

15 Increasing activity is a great way of getting out and about whilst also burning calories, keeping fit and improving circulation. As a guide, the government recommends that we all engage in at least 30 minutes of moderate activity for a minimum of 5 days a week. This need not be taken in one go; 3 ten-minute bouts of activity a day is just as good. Children are more likely to engage in physical activity if at least one of their parents is active so there is an added incentive for you to get active together.

16 Here are some simple ideas to get you and your kids up and about:

- Get out the karaoke machine or buy a dance mat and have a boogie for hours of active fun in your lounge!
- Take the kids to the park and play footie, frisbee or tag, or head out to the water park, fun park or beach.
- Encourage your children to get involved in a hobby they enjoy – they needn't be sporty ones – even painting, drama or music will keep them away from their PCs and the telly; they'll be less likely to snack, learn something new and it will keep you on your toes taking them to the classes or events. For older kids, why not try paintballing, assault courses or dancing classes?
- Walk the kids to school – they'll love you for it, and so will your partner!
- Go for a bike ride or take the kids roller blading, skate boarding or ice-skating and show them what a big kid you really are!
- Get the kids to help you wash the car or help out in the garden. Set up a rota for the housework or the washing up. Kids need to see both parents taking responsibility for household chores.
- Book an active holiday not a week lounging on the beach.
- Consider having a dog in the family – but only if you're ready to be responsible for their weight and health, too.
- Have a TV-free day each week.
- Enter the family in a local fun-run and train for it together – It'll bring out everyone's competitive streak and be a real incentive to get out of the house, even if it's cold and dark!

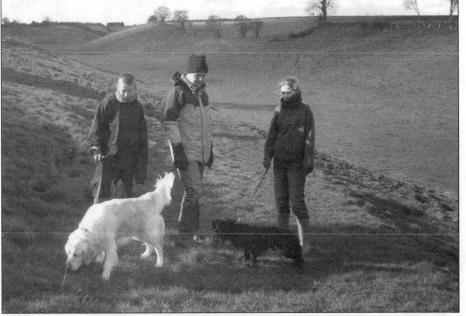

Consider having a dog (or two) in the family – but only if you're ready to be responsible for their weight and health, too!

5 Fat Facts

Statistics

• A child who is obese by 12 years of age has an 80% chance of becoming an obese adult.

• Obesity in young adult life will lower your life expectancy by 5-20 yrs.

• Children who spend more than 5 hours a day watching television are 8 times more likely to become obese.

1 Excessive attempts to control children's eating habits are linked to weight gain – perhaps because children never learn to recognise their own internal sense of hunger and fullness.

2 Girls who have fathers who support their activities are more physically active than those who are not.

Myths

Obese children have a low metabolism

There is no evidence to suggest that fatter people have a low metabolism. In fact, studies have shown that the number of calories used by the body during periods of rest actually increases as children become fatter, ie, the larger you are, the more calories your body uses.

Low in fat = low calories

Don't make the assumption that a low-fat food is also low in calories. For example, a chocolate bar might be 98% fat free but yet be loaded with sugar and calories. The best way to work out the calorie content of a food is to look at the nutrition panel on the product. Information per 100g of product allows you to compare the nutritional content of one food against another.

Fat children are happy children

Children who are overweight or obese may be seen as content children but in reality, they may be labelled as ugly and lazy and be unpopular with their peers. You may remember the fat child in the class being the last to be picked for school sports teams. These children can become depressed and develop a low self-esteem.

Strange but true

• People who consume bigger portions do not necessarily feel fuller for longer than those who consume smaller portions of the same foods.

• Foods rich in fat make you eat more.

• Snacking in itself is not associated with obesity. Studies have shown that it is the type of foods that are eaten, rather than the action of snacking itself, that is linked to weight gain.

• Kids who lie in could be doing themselves good! Research shows that kids who sleep for longer tend to be slimmer than those that rise early. Possible explanations are that this reduces the time available to eat, that sleeping affects their hormones (and therefore their appetite) or that they are less tired during their waking hours and therefore more active than early risers.

• Obese adults who were obese as children find it harder to lose weight than those that were slim as kids so there's an added incentive to take action now.

6 Instructor's section for fathers

"My kids help me lose weight already – they cause me constant stress and worry and take all my money"
(Jack Knife, father of two)

1 Once you've mastered HGV, you have a duty to pass on this knowledge to learner drivers. This section is for those HGV licence-holders with responsibilities for instruction and maintenance of mini HGVs. We consider key issues for safe and effective instruction.

2 Within this are considered methods of developing team dynamics to assist optimum vehicle performance. Most of these may be less traumatic than those techniques experienced by Mr Knife.

Preparing for instruction

3 Effective instruction requires a motivated and energetic instructor, as well as a motivated and energetic learner. Here are some tips to help achieve this...

Take on more fuel!

4 To keep up with your kids, you'll need to maintain high energy levels. Try introducing a bowl of porridge with fruit at breakfast. This should provide you with more energy in the afternoon. You may also find that there is no longer a trigger telling you either to snack excessively between meals or pig-out at the evening meal. Without even trying to lose weight (you were more interested in the extra energy) you've lost a few pounds along the way.

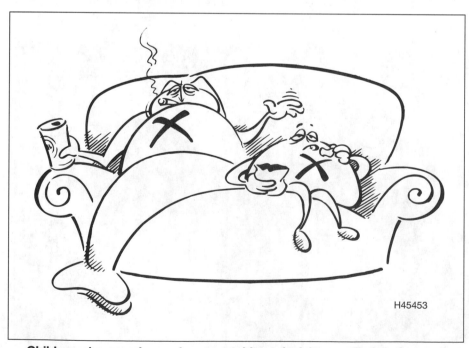

H45453

Children who spend many hours watching television are likely to become obese

Recruiting mini HGVs

5 Usually, kids are interested in health. The health of family members provides an abundance of topic areas for meal-time discussions. Children love to gain knowledge about and to contribute in the process of keeping family members healthy. The truth is, they're ready for recruitment the moment you're ready to instruct. Once they're on board, team tactics can be developed. These can be much more effective than driving solo.

Learners need rest

6 Remember that when the kids get back from school they're almost certainly just as fragile and short-tempered as you are when you get back from work. They need space, quiet time. Then they'll recoup their energies and be ready for the tutorial.

Model driver

7 As a dad you may recall the eating and exercise habits of your own father. These will inevitably have influenced how you now eat and drink. Now you're in that role. You eat sensibly – the kids eat sensibly. You exercise regularly, the kids exercise regularly. Remember your offspring will at some point inevitably make an assessment of you as a person they want to be like or a person they may want to know, even marry. Clearly you won't want a slob as a relative.

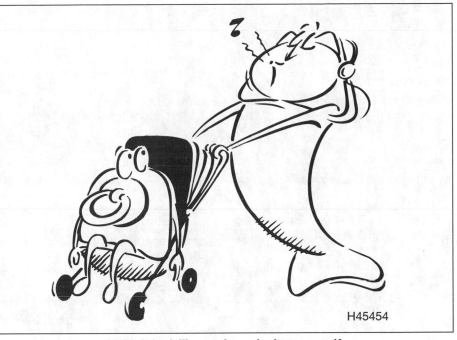

H45454

Make it look like you're enjoying yourself

Enjoy yourself

8 The most important message for your kids is that they see you *enjoying* your lifestyle. If you're not enjoying what you're doing, guaranteed the kids will pick this up and no-one will enjoy it. So the healthy choices you make need to be ones that keep you feeling good. The same goes for when you're involving the kids – it needs to be something that you can all get something from. For example, if you're being asked to play football in the garden, fine – as long as you get your choice of music.

Remember – you're a hero

9 Hollywood has much to blame for the portrayal of heroes as macho beer-swigging womanisers. However, where the movie-makers often do get it right is that the good guy is usually active,

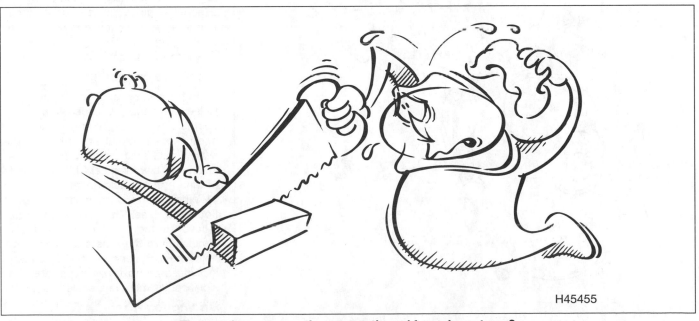

H45455

The good guys are active, energetic and fun; why not you?

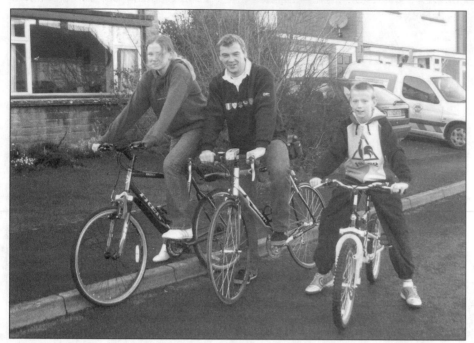

Go out for a cycle ride with the children (but don't forget the helmets!)

energetic and fun. These are the ideal characteristics of a father as a healthy role model.

Maintain your independence

10 Over time, poor diet and exercise will inevitably take its toll on your body and mean you will rely more on others – Doctors, partners, etc (don't you just hate relying on others for anything?!). Sensible diet and exercise will help you retain independence, staving off reliance on others. Think about it…. Your kids see you maintain your independence.

They'll see you value this, value it themselves and work towards the same. Chances are they'll then be out of your house and out of your hair that bit sooner. Remember, if you don't take control, your kids will think it's okay to be lazy and end up relying on you for longer.

Effective Instruction

11 First, let's consider things that some consider to be effective instruction, but which aren't…

- *Instructor and learner lifting cans of drinks to lips in unison.*
- *Simultaneously moving to retrieve TV remote control from coffee table.*
- *Watching every screened football match on TV.*
- *A family meal out: pizza and chips.*

12 Whereas, effective instruction might include:

- *Playing football in the park at weekends.*
- *Going for a cycle ride together an a summer's evening.*
- *Sharing responsibilities for barbeques of chicken and salad.*
- *Walking together two evenings a week.*
- *Taking turns to cook porridge in the mornings.*

Instruction about appetite

13 Learner drivers need to understand the basics about weight management, and more often than not, it's about appetite control. Using the right fuel at regular intervals (eg, 3 main meals and 3 snacks) gives greater control over appetite and is essential to avoid overloading. This message is really worth stressing to learners.

When they're young

14 Pram walks can be dull. You've got to feel good about the occasion. Provide yourself with an incentive. Make a beeline for a pub that's about 20 minutes away. Fresh air and the promise of a pub lunch (say a wholemeal BLT and a glass of wine) – that should do it.

15 When you're walking, do your pelvic floor exercises. This will not only help relieve boredom, but also boosts circulation to the prostate (important to help prevent cancer), and because it increases blood-flow to that area, can significantly improve erectile function!

Driving together

16 You don't have to spend every

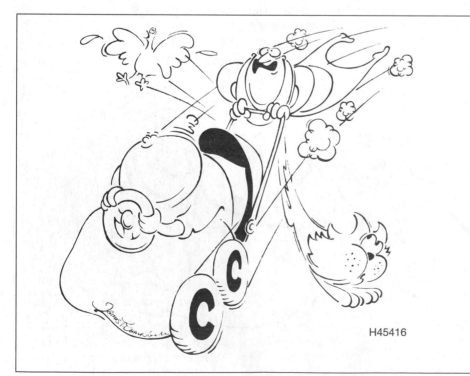

H45416

Pram walks don't have to be totally dull

weekend on walking expeditions together in the Pennines. Much better is a 20 minute walk to the shops during the week, or an hour in the park on a Saturday with a football.

17 Say it's 7 o'clock in the evening. You've all had your tea, Coronation Street doesn't start for half-an-hour and there's certainly nothing worth watching until then. Okay, so you've been told you need a pint of milk for the morning (semi-skimmed of course). Now you could ask the oldest child to make the two-minute walk to the newsagent's. Or you could drive yourself. Or you could suggest that the you and one of the kids go together and aim for the supermarket, which is a bit further, a 20-minute round walk. One of these options will give you the chance for some quality time with your sprog, as well as giving you both some exercise. "But what if it's raining?" Umbrella and boots make it a bit more of an adventure (for the kids, of course, not you, you wuss)!

The new trucker's breakfast

18 On a Saturday morning, why not treat yourself and the kids to a proper English 'trucker's' breakfast? Poached egg, grilled back bacon, tomato, and microwaved mushrooms on wholemeal bread, accompanied by a glass of orange juice.

Understanding women drivers

19 As boys ourselves, we can be ill-equipped to know what motivates girls to buy into this sensible diet and exercise stuff. You may well need to spend additional time talking with the female learners to find out where they're at.

Music

20 Music is a cheap and entertaining way of keeping fit. How does that work, you may ask. Well at the very least it's a distraction from eating. Once you start strumming a guitar or singing, time tends to pass pretty fast, and before you know it you've spent a couple of hours with no thought about re-fuelling.

Fuel preparation

21 Cooking is one of the most pleasing activities in which to involve kids. There's nothing like filling the kitchen with the fragrance of homemade oatmeal biscuits. Also, you'll be amazed at how

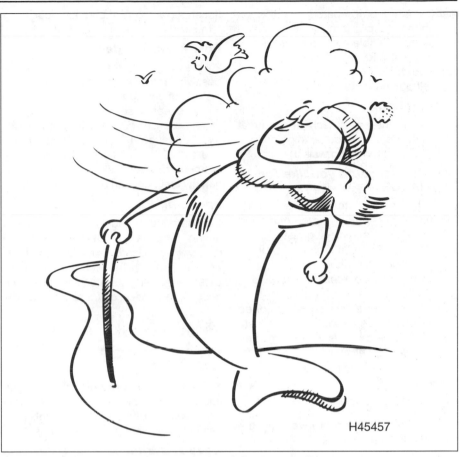

H45457

Nothing on telly? Go for a walk

Distraction tip – what about a guitar?

Do you know any Beatles' songs? The kids might know one or two. The guitar is a cool instrument, and you don't have to be Eric Clapton to become a pretty competent player. A second-hand guitar can be bought for about £30, and once you've bought a couple of good music books, there is very little on-going additional cost. There are some good Beatles guitar books out there. Get some advice, but you'll find that most of these start with simple stuff and move on to the more complex pieces, but the beauty of this is you learn at your own rate. If there's someone you know who plays already – they'll be a help, but with the right book you'll be amazed at how quickly you get going with it and the kids'll be well impressed. Even just 10 minutes a day – you'll be strumming Yellow Submarine in a fortnight. Once you've mastered Beatles, the rest will follow. At Christmas time, carols are easy to master and are a must.

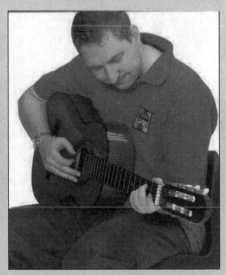

Making music takes your mind off food, at the very least

many kids will be prepared to make you a packed lunch (say a ham salad sandwich on wholemeal bread) for just a couple of quid. You may even be tempted to have a go at preparing it yourself on occasions.

Braking habits

22 Walking the kids to school is a great start to the day. If it's too far to go on foot, try parking half-way and walk the rest.

Dad – what would you like for Christmas?

23 Birthdays, Christmas, Easter... Kids love giving presents, but are often short of ideas. Here are some suggestions:

- *A decent umbrella (for the evening walks if you've wimped out!).*
- *A good book (to keep you outside in the summer).*
- *Bags of whole almonds or dried apricots (for your snacks – both taste great, provide loads of energy and have a good shelf life).*
- *Packs of sugar free gum (to have when driving).*

Washing the car

24 Get the kids out there washing the car with you (not for you).

Indoor workouts

25 If you use gym equipment in the house, or video workouts are your thing – the kids will love to join in with this.

Positive messages

26 It's a good idea to focus on the positive aspects of dieting. For example, instead of saying to the learner, that you need to eat a sensible breakfast and lunch because you "need to lose weight". try, "because I want to have more energy". Older kids can be particularly concerned about skin condition – a healthy diet here can really help.

Speeding fine

27 Someone needs to step in if you're falling into bad habits – eating too quickly, too much or exercising too little. Try employing the learner as your personal trainer – they can fine you on the spot. Great motivation for all concerned!

---

7   How to... control appetite

1 Snacks of fruit or nuts mid-morning, mid-afternoon and evening will help you keep your appetite under control, thus helping to prevent pig-out sessions.

Have you tried?

- For more energy – a glass of water!
- Balsamic vinegar as an alternative to salad dressing – just as tasty, but no fat!
- Drinking a large glass of water a few minutes before a meal – feel full earlier, with no extra calories!
- Time for a leak? It's easy to go to the nearest lav when you're at work. But how about stretching your legs a bit more and finding the loo furthest away in the building. Do this a couple of times each day and you'll be clocking up towards target for daily steps.

---

8   Strange but true

- Many children who skip breakfast are significantly heavier than those who eat breakfast...

Australian Government publication, 2004

- People who eat breakfast have more nutritious diets than people who skip breakfast and have better eating habits as they are less likely to be hungry for snacks during the day.

Australian Government publication, 2004

- Remember: Eat, drink and be merry, for tomorrow you may live!
- Some eye specialists feel that it won't be eyesight that suffers as much as the increased risk of obesity and poor posture that comes from excessive use of computers. Make sure you spend 15 minutes away from the computer each hour – do some stretching exercises instead.

---

9   That Middle Age Spread... Obesity and Older Men

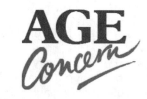

Introduction

"I have been overweight for most of my life... I feel that my fat is a wall to bounce the world off. I know that the weight I carry is not good for my health. I know that I overeat out of habit and a need for comfort. It is the only way I allow myself to look after me. I have now... started to lose weight. I believe that what is

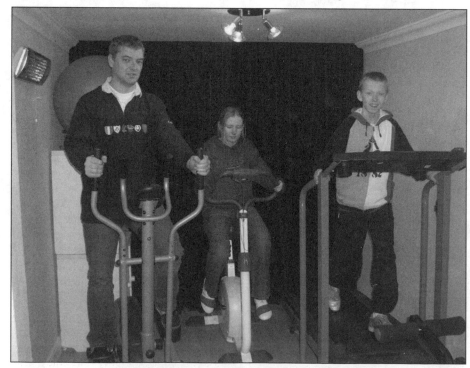

If you've got a home gym, use it as a family

enabling me to change is that I am now looking after the upset part of me to a greater extent. Both through being in a men's group and through co-counselling, I am feeling rather than suppressing the hurts in my life. I am softening the stiff upper lip." Jonk Watts[1]

1 Statistics show that obesity increases with age. Recent statistics show that about 27% of men and 31% of women ages 16-24 are overweight or obese, but these figures rise to 79% for men and 71% of women aged 55-64.[2]

2 In many respects, older men today live in a different world from that of their fathers. The reduction in physical work in their daily lives has made a significant contribution to the recent epidemic of obesity. Overweight/obesity is now the most widespread and rapidly increasing nutritional disorder in the developed world.

3 Modern lifestyles make it very easy for individuals to be inactive. More men are eating convenience or junk food and only 20 percent of older men take light to moderate exercise (e.g. golf, cycling, and brisk walks).[3] Time spent watching television is also directly proportional to the risk of obesity.

4 Obesity reduces life expectancy by, on average, nine years.[4]

Older men and attitudes towards general healthcare

5 Research has shown that many older men are unwilling to contact health professionals in later life. Whilst women have routinely visited their GP surgeries throughout their lives for contraception, pregnancy or with their children, men are reluctant to go to the doctor and see it as a sign of weakness. Often they do not want to be seen to *give in* to sickness, and admit to postponing making an appointment until they are very sick. Such delays can have obvious long term adverse health consequences.

Causes of obesity in older men

6 The causes of overweight/obesity can often be simplified into three components: diet, physical activity and genes which determine individual predisposition to effects on appetite and metabolism. It is clear that obesity runs in families, is more common in some ethnic groups and is seen more frequently in developed countries where there is an analogy between socioeconomic status and obesity.

7 Obesity tends to run in families and this could be explained by environmental factors given that families often share the same diet, lifestyle and cultural influences. These habits tend to persist into later life.

Prevalence of Obesity

Partnership status

8 The partnership status of older men has been found to have an impact on their health and by extension their levels of obesity. Poor diets and levels of alcohol consumption are higher in men who are widowed or divorced.[5]

9 Membership of sports and social clubs declines significantly with age. Widowers are more involved with sports and social clubs than married men, perhaps indicating that leisure associations offer compensations following widowhood. Divorced and never married older men have very low involvement in organisations.[6]

Socio-economic status

10 There is proven association between material disadvantage and poor health in later life. The major factors associated with older men smoking, having a poor diet and taking little physical activity are the class of their last occupation, living on a low income and living in more materially deprived circumstances. The highest levels of excessive drinking are found among the most deprived and socially isolated older men.[7]

11 Some older men do not always have the means to change health-related behaviour to choose healthy foods, for example, because of their incomes. A report produced by Age Concern[8] shows that nearly half of all pensioners and as many as 80% of those who are local authority tenants do not receive a decent income (£160.00 a week for homeowners and £200 for tenants).

Diet

12 The average household diet in Britain has changed dramatically since the last war. Since the austere days of rationing

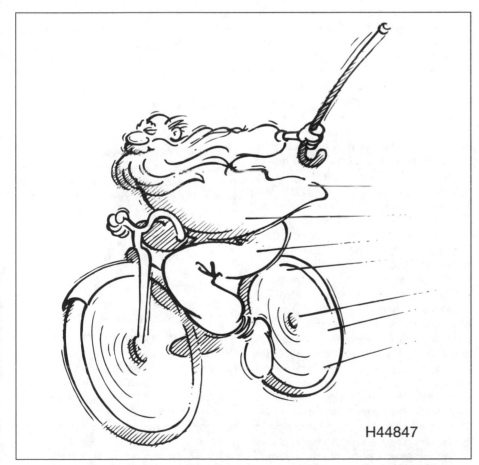

H44847

Physical activity is very important in maintaining overall good health

there have been widespread changes – all of which have had a major impact on what people eat today. There has been a large increase in ready-prepared, convenience, and fast foods.

13 All fast foods are of low nutritional value and are low in vitamins and minerals which are required to keep people healthy. Instead they provide large amounts of calories and fat, which can contribute to weight gain.

14 Healthy eating is important throughout life. As well as obesity, many chronic diseases that develop in later life, such as osteoporosis, can be influenced by poor habits in earlier life. Good nutrition in later life, however, can still help lessen the effects of disease prevalent amongst older people, or significantly improve the quality of life in people who have such diseases. It is never too late to change eating and other habits, in order to lose weight and maintain higher levels of health and vitality which, in turn, can make life more enjoyable.

15 Nutritionists agree that the basis of a healthy diet should be:

- *To eat a variety of foods.*
- *To eat more foods rich in starch and fibre – especially cereal foods, vegetables and fruit.*
- *To eat fewer fatty foods.*
- *To cut down on sugary foods.*
- *To drink alcohol only in moderation.*

Physical Activity

16 Many older people who are obese are also inactive. It should not therefore be a surprise to older men that long periods of sedentary living can lead to serious health problems. People who are sedentary double their risk of premature death and run the risk of suffering from problems such as heart disease, diabetes, some cancers as well as obesity. In addition, regular activity can help alleviate other risk factors such as high blood pressure and unhealthy blood fats.

17 The reduction in physical work in people's lives has made a considerable contribution to the recent epidemic of obesity. To counteract this, people need to use up more energy through walking, climbing, lifting and pushing as they go about their household and occupational chores. Small changes in routine such as taking the stairs, walking to the shops and washing the car manually can increase energy expenditure over the week and contribute to weight management.

18 Physical activity is very important in helping to maintain not only a healthy weight but in maintaining overall good health. There is increasing evidence of the benefits of physical activity in relation to disease prevention, mobility, independence and quality of life. Despite the increase in the promotion of exercise and physical activity for prevention of functional decline and disease, people in the UK become less physically active as they age.[9]

Obesity and other health problems

19 Older age greatly increases the risk of diabetes, joint disorders, breathing difficulties and possibly motility. Prevention is always better than cure, and an important aspect of health promotion in the 'younger' older people is to maintain a healthy weight. This can become difficult, however, especially as physical activity levels decline.

20 For those who do become overweight, strict dieting is not advised in later life, as this reduces the intake of essential nutrients. Instead, the balance of food intakes should be changed, reducing sugary and fatty foods, while increasing bread, cereals, fruits and vegetables. Increasing the amount of regular, gentle exercise will also help achieve slow, sensible weight loss.

21 The young elderly may have 20 or so active years ahead of them, so health promotion and fitness are the primary aims when it comes to nutrition. The older elderly are more likely to develop chronic illnesses, which will probably be coupled with the need for more support. This age group is the fastest growing sector in society and has specific nutritional needs. However, nutritional advice should be based on individual needs rather than chronological age.

22 A recent Government report, *The Diet and Nutritional Survey of People Aged 65 Years and Over*, showed that older people in the UK are generally adequately nourished. However, on further investigation, the results show a mixed pattern of nutritional status. While 60 per cent of men and women living in the community were overweight, those living in residential or nursing homes were more likely to be underweight (one in six), deficient in folate (a B vitamin) or anaemic.

23 A much more common link between excess weight and metabolic disease is diabetes. Middle-aged and elderly people who are overweight are far more likely to develop type II, non-insulin dependent, diabetes. Often, merely shedding the excess weight leads to good control of the disease. Diabetes is a serious condition, which significantly increases the risk of coronary heart disease and stroke.

Using Age Concern to help you lose weight

24 Many Age Concerns provide activities which can help you to lose weight – for example Age Concern Surrey has walking groups, cycling groups and gym sessions especially for the over 50s.

25 If you don't fancy 'exercise' then why not try dancing yourself slimmer? Many Age Concerns have regular tea dances, which as well as being good exercise, also provide an opportunity for you to socialise and meet new people.

26 Age Concern recognises that making healthy choices is difficult if you are worried about money or other issues. Most Age Concerns have 'information and advice' services to help you deal with these issues.

Using 'Ageing Well UK' to help you lose weight

27 Some Age Concerns run 'Ageing Well' programmes where older volunteers are recruited and trained to become 'Senior Health Mentors'. These mentors work with their local communities to give health promotion advice to their peers. This advice ranges from 'healthy cooking for one' courses to 'physical activity motivating' – where a mentor will work with older people one-to-one to help them take more exercise. There are over 100 'Ageing Well' projects in the UK

Using your grandchildren to help you lose weight

28 Many older people report that they want to stay fit and healthy in order to see their grandchildren grow up and allow them to play together.

29 Spend time playing with your grandchildren – a 'kick-about' in the park with the children can use up calories and is cheaper than going to the gym!

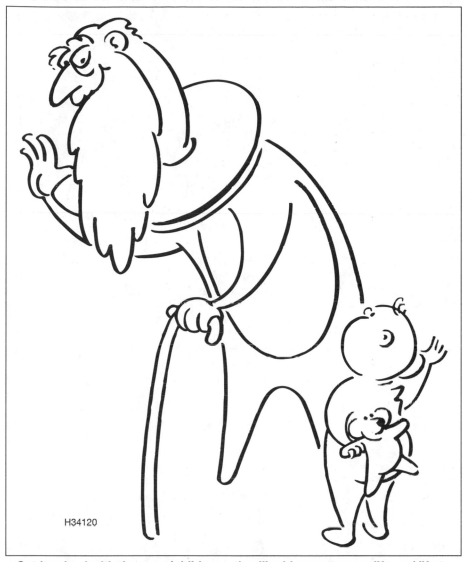

Get involved with the grandchildren – they'll add years to your life and life to your years.

30 Many children love learning about how things grow – teach your grandchildren gardening techniques and grow some healthy fruit and vegetables together, then enjoy eating the results! You don't have to have an allotment or large vegetable patch, salad vegetables can be grown in small containers.

Conclusion

31 The availability of food, especially those with a high fat content, and the ease with which physical activity can be avoided prevent many older men from making the changes which are needed to reduce their weight or maintain a healthy weight in older age. Combining an active lifestyle with a healthy, balanced diet will help older men to:

- *Stay in shape.*
- *Feel fitter and have more energy.*
- *Keep the digestive system regular.*
- *Increase concentration and optimise memory and mood.*
- *Support the immune system to keep infections at bay and recover more quickly from an illness.*
- *Reduce the risk of health problems like obesity and osteoporosis.*
- *Add 'years to life and life to years'.*

Further information

32 If you would like to know more, look in the Contacts section at the back of the book, or contact:

Age Concern England
Astral House
1268 London Road
London
SW16 4ER
Tel: 020 8765 7200
Information Line: 0800 00 99 66
Fax: 020 8765 7211
Website: www.ageconcern.org.uk

References

1 Bruckenwell. P., Jackson. D., Luck. M., Wallace., J., Watts, J. 1995. *The Crisis in Men's Health.* Community Health, UK.
2 British Heart Foundation – http://www.bhf.org.uk/questions – 2004
3 British Heart Foundation – Factfile 07/99
4 Weight Concern. 2004. *What does it matter if someone is overweight or obese?* www.shape-up.org/weightcon/matter.html
5 Arber, A & Davidson, K. 2003. *Older Men: Their Social Worlds and Healthy Lifestyles.* ESRC Growing Older Programme – Research Findings:12.
6 Ibid.
7 Cooper, H., Ginn, J. & Arber, S. 1999. *Health-related behaviour and attitudes of older people.* Health Education Authority.
8 Age Concern. 2002. *Modest but Adequate*
9 Skelton, D & Dinan, S. 1999. *Exercise for falls management: Rationale for an exercise programme to reduce postural instability.* Physiotherapy : Theory & Practice; 15:105-20.

Contents

WEIGHT ON THE WEB

By Jim Pollard

1 The internet is getting very, very fat. Google, the most-used search engine, includes as many as four billion pages and even that's less than half of the searchable web! Where do you start?

2 What you'll want to know depends on who you are. The information needs of someone who is overweight will be different from those of someone who has just been diagnosed with an eating disorder or weight-related health problem, the needs of someone who wants basic nutritional information different from those of someone with an allergy, the needs of a parent worried about a child different from those of a health professional.

3 To use the internet to find out what you want to know takes time and a little knowledge about how internet search engines work.

4 The first thing to note is that despite their name, internet search engines do not actually search the internet. They search their own databases which in turn link to real websites. Search engines use programs called spiders to check these links from time to time but they are not always up to date. That's why you sometimes click on a link on a search engine to a page that is no longer there.

5 Spiders find new pages to add to their database by going to the pages they already know about and following the links from those pages. In other words, if a page is not linked to any other, a spider cannot find it. An unlinked site will only appear on a search engine if it has been submitted to it directly. (Google and all search engines offer this facility.)

6 Search engine statistics are staggering. There are 250 million searches on Google every day. Do a Google search on 'food' and you'll get 213,000,000 results. Refine that to 'diet' and you'll get 43,600,000. Opt for 'Atkins', the most recent in a long, long list of fad diets, and you'll still get over nine million. 'Obesity' gets a similar score. Where do you start? The top of the list? Not necessarily.

7 Spiders rely on links to find new sites. Search engines use a similar system to govern where on a search a particular site appears. Generally speaking, the more links, the higher the ranking. The theory is that the number of links reflects the popularity and so the usefulness of that site. This sounds fine in theory but may simply mean that the website has included as many links as possible and never mind the quality or relevance. Many commercial sites have long lists of so-called 'links'. The Men's Health Forum website, for example, is inundated with proposed link 'exchanges', many from wholly unsuitable sites. The Forum rarely says yes. But the reality is that if they did they'd probably feature even higher on web searches.

8 Search engines also tend to prioritise sites which are selling something rather than those offering merely information – a big problem with a controversial subject like diet and weight where there's money to be made.

9 Is the organisation running the site you're looking at reliable? Many sites have an About Us section which you can check out. If you don't know who they are, be wary. Is the site simply a shop window or part of the marketing of a product or does it aim to provide information for its own sake? Unless stated, all the sites listed below are in the second group. Approach those in the first group with care.

10 Refine your search. The only good thing that you can say about 230,000,000 pages on 'food' is that at least reading them all will stop you eating, probably for several months.

11 To get the best out of a search engine, try to be specific. Use the 'advanced search' option if available. This may allow you to select only UK sites or only those updated in, say, the last three months. This is not because you are only interested in new information but because you may want to avoid dormant sites which are no longer being updated.

12 You aren't restricted to searching for individual words. You can use speech marks to search for specific phrases. For example, to search for "metabolic syndrome". Also use + (plus) and - (minus/dash) to narrow down your results. For example: 'diabetes +weight-loss' will retrieve items that mention both diabetes and weight-loss. The minus command might help if, for example, you wanted to find research by your doctor, the unfortunately named Dr Jekyll, but didn't want to be inundated with Robert Louis Stevenson references. You could try "Dr Jekyll" -"Mr Hyde".

13 A combination of the above can be very powerful indeed, enabling pinpoint searches. For example, "metabolic syndrome" +"Dr Jekyll" +"Belchester Bugle" could help you to track down that article your friend reckoned he'd seen in his local paper about your doctor and metabolic syndrome. This assumes, of course, that your search engine is aware of the Belchester Bugle website which, as we've already seen, is far from guaranteed.

14 Although most search engines recognise short-cuts like pluses and minuses, not all engines work in the same way so a bit of trial and error is needed to get the best out of them. (Search engines within a particular site – rather than a global search engine like Google – can be particularly frustrating as they are frequently built on far simpler technology.)

15 Get a second opinion. Not only do search engines all work differently, they also all include different content. Many, many pages appear only on one search engine and no other so it's always worth getting a second or third opinion. At the time of writing, malehealth.co.uk had 230 links to it on Google, compared with 929 on altavista.com and 951 on yahoo.co.uk.

16 So should you use the web to find advice on diet and weight? Yes, but be careful. As you will have learned from this book, although it's possible to give general nutritional guidelines for most people in most situations, a diet needs to be customised to the individual. That's where the health professional comes in. The internet is a resource that can help you get the most from a consultation with a nutritionist, practice nurse, doctor, or qualified local health club or gym coach. But it is not a substitute for a professional consultation.

17 Don't underestimate the value of the net. Simply remember that you use it at your own risk. *All these websites are listed for information only and neither the author nor the publishers can accept any responsibility for their content.*

Starting points

18 See Contacts for website addresses.

Other interesting links

19 If your diet is such that you're primarily interested in the facts about fast food and health, try this link from the office of the Attorney General for Minnesota in the USA: **www.olen.com/food/book.html**

20 Another good briefing on the same subject, but a bit more difficult to type in, is **www.mrc.ac.uk/index/public-interest/public-news-4/public-news_archive/public-news-archive_oct_03/public-fast_food.htm**

21 Meanwhile, the interactive questionnaire run by the Center for Science in the Public Interest in the US will tell you exactly how healthy your restaurant food choices are: **www.cspinet.org/nah/quiz/index.html**

22 If you're after greater details on the value or otherwise of your entire daily diet, you'll want this site, run by the US Department of Agriculture Center for Nutrition Policy and Promotion (**209.48.219.53**). It lets users analyse their personal daily food intake, including total fat, saturated fat, cholesterol, and sodium.

23 For recipes that might help, try: **www.fatfreekitchen.com/**

24 It can be harder to eat a healthy diet on a low income. The Food for Thought section of the Oxford Brookes University site is aimed at students but contains healthy eating tips for anyone on budget: **cs3.brookes.ac.uk/student/services/health/food.html**

25 For younger readers, the Health Development Agency has set up some excellent sites. Welltown (**www.welltown.gov.uk**) is for teachers and children at key stage 1 (ages 5-7). Galaxy H (**www.galaxy-h.gov.uk**) is for key stage 2 (ages 7-11). LifeBytes (**www.lifebytes.gov.uk**) for key stage 3 (ages 11-14) includes a good section on healthy eating. As does Mind, Body & Soul (**www.mindbodysoul.gov.uk**) which is for key stage 4 (ages 14-16).

26 A good introduction to the glycemic index is at **www.glycemicindex.com/** which is a system of ranking of carbohydrates based on their immediate effect on blood glucose (blood sugar) levels. The link **diabetes.about.com/library/mendosagi/ngilists.htm** provides a straight-forward glycemic table of 750 foods.

27 And finally, if after all this you need more links, **www.diet-links.com/** has dozens of them.

Contacts

Action for Leisure
Promotes play and leisure with and for disabled adults and children.
PO Box 9
West Molesey
KT8 1WT
Tel: 020 8783 0173
Fax: 020 8783 9267
e-mail: enquiries@actionforleisure.org.uk
Website: www.actionforleisure.org.uk

Action on Smoking and Health (ASH)
ASH is a campaigning public health charity working for a comprehensive societal response to tobacco aimed at achieving a sharp reduction and eventual elimination of the health problems caused by tobacco. 120,000 people per year die from smoking-related diseases in the UK and tobacco is a major cause of illness and health inequalities. Tobacco is a powerfully addictive drug that most of its users would like to quit using.
102 Clifton Street
London
EC2A 4HW
Tel: 020 7739 5902
Fax: 020 7613 0531
e-mail: enquiries@ash.org.uk
Website: www.ash.org.uk

Action on Smoking and Health (ASH) Scotland
ASH Scotland is the leading voluntary organisation in Scotland tackling tobacco use. Established in 1973, the organisation holds a wealth of experience and knowledge on tobacco issues.
8 Frederick Street
Edinburgh
EH2 2HB
Tel: 0131 225 4725
Fax: 0131 225 4759
e-mail: ashscotland@ashscotland.org.uk
Website: www.ashscotland.org.uk

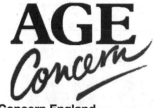

Age Concern England
Age Concern supports all people over 50 in the UK, ensuring that they get the most from life. We provide essential services such as day care and information. We campaign on issues like age discrimination and pensions, and work to influence public opinion and government policy about older people.
Astral House
1268 London Road
London , SW16 4ER
Tel: 020 8765 7200
Information Line: 0800 00 99 66
Fax: 020 8765 7211
Website: www.ageconcern.org.uk

Aikido UK
33 Owen Avenue
Murray 12
East Kilbride, G75 9AH
Tel: 01355 220419
e-mail: aikidouk@hotmail.com
Website: www.aikido-uk.org

Alcohol Concern
Alcohol Concern is the national agency on alcohol misuse. We work to reduce the incidence and costs of alcohol-related harm and to increase the range and quality of services available to people with alcohol-related problems.
Waterbridge House
32-36 Loman Street
London
SE1 0EE
Tel: 020 7928 7377
Fax: 020 7928 4644
e-mail: contact@alcoholconcern.org.uk
Website: www.alcoholconcern.org.uk/

Alcohol unit calculator
Website: www.projects.ex.ac.uk/trol/scol/ccalcoh2.htm

Alcoholics Anonymous
Tel: 0845 769 7555 (local rate calls)

Amateur Rowing Association
The ARA is the governing body for the sport of rowing in England, and is also responsible for representing Great Britain's interests to FISA, and for the preparation, training and selection of GB teams. At a national level the ARA is also responsible for the organisation and development of rowing in England.
6 Lower Mall
Hammersmith
London
W6 9DJ
Tel: 020 8237 6700
Fax: 020 8237 6749
e-mail: info@ara-rowing.org
Website: www.ara-rowing.org

Amateur Swimming Association (ASA)
The Amateur Swimming Association is the English national governing body for swimming, diving, water polo, open water and synchronised swimming. The ASA aims to ensure everybody has an opportunity to learn to swim.
Harold Fern House
Derby Square
Loughborough
Leicestershire
LE11 5AL
Tel: 01509 618 700
Fax: 01509 618 701
e-mail:
customerservices@swimming.org
Website: www.britishswimming.org

American Heart Association
What constitutes a good basic diet?
Website: www.americanheart.org/presenter.jhtml?identifier=4561

American Obesity Association
The site of a leading US organisation in the field. They reckon it's the 'most comprehensive site on obesity and overweight on the internet'.
Website: www.obesity.org

Anorexia and Bulimia Care (ABC)
Anorexia and Bulimia Care (ABC) has been in existence in its present form since 1989. It is a national Christian organisation run by Christians for sufferers, their families and for carers.
PO Box 173
Letchworth
Hertfordshire, SG6 1XQ
Tel: 01462 423351
e-mail:
anorexiabulimiacare@ntlworld.com
Website:
www.anorexiabulimiacare.co.uk

Archery
Websites: www.gnas.org or
www.nfas.net

Arthritis Care
Arthritis Care is the UK's largest voluntary organisation working with and for people with arthritis. We aim to empower people to take control of their arthritis and their lives.
18 Stephenson Way
London , NW1 2HD
Tel: 020 7380 6500 (general enquiries)
Fax: 020 7380 6505
e-mail: helplines@arthritiscare.org.uk
Website: www.arthritiscare.org.uk

The Arthritis Foundation of Ireland
The Arthritis Foundation of Ireland was established in 1981. It is the only national charity dedicated to further Research and Education for this common condition. The Foundation is continuing to fund research into arthritis in Ireland. The long term aim is to find a cure for the disease but along the way research projects funded increase our understanding of the disease and so improve treatment given.
1 ClanWilliam Square
Grand Canal Quay
Dublin 2
Ireland
Tel: 01 6618188
Fax: 01 661 6261
e-mail: info@arthritis-foundation.com
Website: www.arthritis-foundation.com

Arthritis Research Campaign (ARC)
The Arthritis Research Campaign (arc), founded in 1936, raises funds to promote medical research into the cause, treatment and cure of arthritic conditions: to educate medical students, doctors and allied healthcare professionals about arthritis and to provide information to people affected by arthritis and to the general public.
Copeman House
St Mary's Court
St Mary's Gate
Chesterfield
Derbyshire
S41 7TD
Tel: 0870 850 5000
Fax: 01246 558007
e-mail: info@arc.org.uk
Website: www.arc.org.uk/

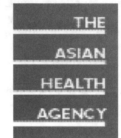

The Asian Health Agency (TAHA)
The Asian Health Agency is a registered charity specialising in the provision of direct and holistic health & social care services and capacity building support services primarily to Asian and other BME communities as well as research, training, consultancy support to statutory and voluntary sectors, particularly in the field of developing culturally appropriate services and anti-discriminatory practices.
Tel: 020 8577 9747
e-mail: admincore@taha.org.uk
Website: www.taha.org.uk

ASSOCIATION FOR THE STUDY OF OBESITY

Association for the Study of Obesity
The Association for the Study of Obesity (ASO) was founded in 1967 and is the UK's foremost organisation dedicated to the understanding and treatment of obesity.

20 Brook Meadow Close
Woodford Green
Essex
London, IG8 9NR
Tel/Fax: 020 8503 2042
e-mail: chris@aso.ndo.co.uk
Website: www.aso.org.uk

Badminton Association of England Ltd
The BAofE is the sport's governing body in England and actively promotes and encourages its development from grass roots, through clubs, local leagues and county organisations to the National Squad.
National Badminton Centre
Bradwell Road
Loughton Lodge
Milton Keynes, MK8 9LA
Tel: 01908 268400
Fax: 01908 268412
e-mail: enquiries@baofe.co.uk
Website: www.baofe.co.uk

Baseball
Tel: 020 7453 7055

BBC Healthy-Living
BBC website with lots of useful information about food and exercise for adults and children. Adults can work out their body mass index (BMI).
Website:
www.bbc.co.uk/health/healthyliving

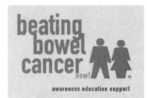

Beating Bowel Cancer
Beating Bowel Cancer is a national charity working to raise awareness of symptoms, promote early diagnosis and encourage open access to treatment choice for those affected by bowel cancer. Through our work we aim to help save lives from this common cancer, the UK's second biggest killer cancer.
39 Crown Road
St. Margarets
Twickenham
Middlesex, TW1 3EJ
Tel: 020 8892 5256
Fax: 020 8892 1008
e-mail info@beatingbowelcancer.org
Website: www.beatingbowelcancer.org

Bikeforall

Cycling is fun, fast, green and healthy. That's why we want you to spend more time pedalling, and less time sitting in front of the computer. Bikeforall.net is a filter, listing the useful bike stuff on the internet, ignoring the duff and the overtly commercial.
Benton Bridge Cottage
Jesmond Dene
Newcastle on Tyne, NE7 7DA
e-mail: editor@bikeforall.net
Website: www.bikeforall.net

Bike Week and Bike2Work National Co-ordinator

Bike Week is the UK's annual promotion of all kinds of cycling. In 2004, more than 180,000 participants in 1,400 events gained a huge amount of positive media coverage for cycling. Funded by the UK governments and the cycle industry's Bike Hub initiative, Bike Week is co-ordinated for a steering group of 16 organisations, all of which want to 'get more people cycling more often'.
10 South Pallant
Chichester, PO19 1SU
Tel: 01243 527444
Mobile: 07730 438082
Fax: 01243 839260
e-mail: nick@bikeweek.org.uk
Website: www.bikeweek.org.uk

Blood Pressure Association

The Blood Pressure Association was established in October 2000 with the aim of making a real difference to the 16 million people affected by high blood pressure in the UK. Our aim at the BPA is to put high blood pressure at the top of everyone's health agenda – from the Government and the media to every adult.
60 Cranmer Terrace
London, SW17 0QS
Tel: 020 8772 4994
Fax: 020 8772 4999
Website: www.bpassoc.org.uk

The Bobby Moore Fund

Raises money for research into bowel cancer and aims to raise awareness of the symptoms so that people are diagnosed earlier.
Cancer Research UK
61 Lincoln's Inn Fields
London, WC2A 3PX
Tel: 020 7269 3412
e-mail: bmf@cancer.org.uk

British Association for Counselling and Psychotherapy

The umbrella membership body for counselling in the UK, and as such the standard-setting association to which all its members adhere, providing support and protection for members of the public who may seek counselling. Provides information on training as a counsellor, as well as information on counselling services available in your locality.
1 Regent Place
Rugby
Warwickshire
CV21 2PJ
Website: www.counselling.co.uk

British Athletics

The British Athletics website has been designed to provide comprehensive, accurate and up to date information on British Athletics.
Umbra Athletics Ltd
Unit 1 Bredbury Business Park
Bredbury Parkway
Bredbury
Stockport
SK6 2SN
Tel: 0161 406 6320
Fax: 0161 406 6732
e-mail: info@britishathletics.info
Website: www.BritishAthletics.Info

British Blind Sport

British Blind Sport is a registered charity and the co-ordinating body of sport for the blind and partially sighted in the UK. The charity was set up in 1975 by visually impaired people, to enable them to have a controlling interest in their various sports.
4-6 Victoria Terrace
Leamington Spa
Warwickshire
CV31 3AB
Tel: 08700 789000
Fax: 08700 789001
email: info@britishblindsport.org.uk
Website: www.britishblindsport.org.uk

The British Cardiac Patients Association

The association offers unconditional help, support, reassurance and advice to cardiac patients, their families and carers. We pride ourselves in being the independent voice of the patient and carer. To that end we represent the patient on Government bodies, research working groups, Health Improvement Programmes, nursing bodies, and many others.
BCPA Head Office
2 Station Road
Swavesey
Cambridge
CB4 5QJ
Tel: 0800 4792800 (freephone)
e-mail: enquiries@BCPA.co.uk
Website: www.bcpa.co.uk/what_is.htm

British Cardiac Society

The British Cardiac Society was established in 1922, and is a charitable body. The majority of our membership are UK cardiologists and cardiac surgeons, but also includes other doctors and healthcare professionals. The Society is involved in education, the setting of clinical standards and research into heart and circulatory diseases.
9 Fitzroy Square
London, W1T 5HW
Tel: 020 7383 3887
e-mail: enquiries@bcs.com
Website: www.bcs.com

The British Council of Disabled People

The British Council of Disabled People is the UK's national organisation of the worldwide Disabled People's Movement. We were set up in 1981 by disabled people to promote our full equality and participation in UK society, and we now represent some 126 groups run by disabled people in the UK at national level.
Litchurch Plaza
Litchurch Lane
Derby
DE24 8AA
Tel: 01332 295551
Fax: 01332 295580
Minicom: 01332 295581
e-mail: general@bcodp.org.uk
Website: www.bcodp.org.uk

British Cycling

The internationally recognised governing body for cycling in Great Britain.
National Cycling Centre
Stuart Street
Manchester
M11 4DQ
Tel: 0870 871 2000
Fax: 0870 871 2001
e-mail: info@britishcycling.org.uk
Website: www.britishcycling.org.uk

British Deaf Sports Council (BDSC)
British Deaf Sports Council (BDSC) was founded in 1930, with the aim of organising competitors to participate in the World Games for the Deaf (now known as Deaflympic), and therefore it is Britain's oldest national sports organisation for a disabled group.
Website:
www.britishdeafsportscouncil.org.uk

The British Dietetic Association
The British Dietetic Association, established in 1936, was formed to provide training and facilities for Dieticians. The Association has developed into a Professional Association that aims to: inform, protect, represent and support.
5th Floor
Charles House
148/9 Great Charles Street
Queensway
Birmingham
B3 3HT
Tel: 0121 200 8080
Fax: 0121 200 8081
e-mail: info@bda.uk.com
Website: www.bda.uk.com/ or www.bdaweightwise.com/bda/

British Egg Information Service (BEIS)
Provides general and nutritional information as well as recipes for eggs.
126-128 Cromwell Road
London
SW7 4ET
Tel: 020 7370 7411
Fax: 020 7373 3926
Website: www.britegg.co.uk

British Ethnic Health Awareness Foundation (BEHAF)
BEHAF is a registered national health awareness trust for community support, health care advice, medical information, and patient's advocacy. Our mission is to promote self-help, healthy eating habits, healthy living styles, and raise health awareness in the wider community.
6 Humber Street
Cheetham Hill
Manchester
M8 0PX
Tel: 0161 281 2888 (Monday-Friday, 9am to 5pm)
e-mail: info@behaf.org.uk
Website: www.behaf.org.uk

British Fencing
1 Baron's Gate
33-35 Rothschild Road
London, W4 5HT
Tel: 020 8742 3032
Fax: 020 8742 3033
e-mail:
british_fencing@compuserve.com
Website: www.britishfencing.com

British Gymnastics
British Gymnastics aims to continually assess, review and meet Gymnastic needs and expectations of our Membership by developing strategies and action plans which embrace best value, challenge current thinking, break down barriers and bring about continuous improvement in Opportunities, Facilities and Competitive results.
Ford Hall
Lilleshall National Sports Centre
Newport
Shropshire
TF10 9NB
Tel: 0845 129 7129
Fax: 0845 1249089
Minicom: 0800 783 7898
e-mail: information@british-gymnastics.org
Website: www.british-gymnastics.org

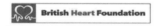

British Heart Foundation
The aim of the British Heart Foundation is to play a leading role in the fight against cardiovascular disease so that it is no longer a major cause of disability and premature death. For more than 40 years, the British Heart Foundation has been at the forefront of the fight against heart disease, funding education, care and much more.
14 Fitzhardinge Street
London , W1H 6DH
Tel: 020 7935 0185
e-mail: internet@bhf.org.uk
Website: www.bhf.org.uk

British Heart Foundation National Centre for Physical Activity and Health (BHFNC)
The British Heart Foundation National Centre for Physical Activity and Health (BHFNC) was established in April 2000 with Funding from the British Heart Foundation (BHF). The BHF continues to fund, support and work in partnership with the Centre.
Loughborough University
Loughborough
Leicestershire
LE11 3TU
Tel: 01509 223259
Fax: 01509 223972
e-mail: bhfactive@lists.lboro.ac.uk
Website: www.bhfactive.org.uk

British Hypertension Society
The British Hypertension Society is a forum for clinicians, physiologists and other scientists with an interest in hypertension. Their website includes details of their meetings, research and publications such as Guidelines for Management of Hypertension.
The Blood Pressure Unit
St. George's Hospital Medical School
Cranmer Terrace
London
SW17 ORE
Tel: 020 8725 3412
Fax: 020 8725 2959
e-mail: bhsis@sghms.ac.uk
Website: www.hyp.ac.uk/bhs

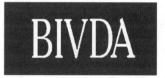

The British In Vitro Diagnostics Association (BIVDA)
The British In Vitro Diagnostics Association (BIVDA) is the national trade association for the In Vitro Diagnostics (IVD) industry.
1 Queen Anne's Gate
London
SW1H 9BT
Website: www.bivda.co.uk

The British Meat Nutrition Education Service
Information on nutrition and the role of lean red meat in a healthy balanced diet.
Good Relations Healthcare
Holborn Gate
26 Southampton Buildings
London
WC2A 1PQ
Tel:; 020 7861 3118
Fax: 020 7861 3913
e-mail: BMNES@grhealthcare.co.uk
Website: www.bmesonline.org.uk

The British Mountaineering Council

The British Mountaineering Council is the representative body that exists to protect the freedoms and promote the interests of climbers, hillwalkers and mountaineers, including ski-mountaineers.
177-179 Burton Rd
Manchester
M20 2BB
Tel: 0870 010 4878
Fax: 0161 445 4500
e-mail: office@thebmc.co.uk
Website: www.thebmc.co.uk/

British Nutrition Foundation

The British Nutrition Foundation is a scientific and educational charity which promotes the well-being of society through the impartial interpretation and effective dissemination of evidence-based nutritional knowledge and advice.
High Holborn House
52-54 High Holborn
London, WC1V 6RQ
Tel: 020 7404 6504
e-mail: postbox@nutrition.org.uk
Website: www.nutrition.org.uk

The British Potato Council

The British Potato Council is all about Improving Competitiveness and Increasing Usage of GB potatoes. We are a non-departmental public body (NDPB) funded by purchasers and growers.
4300 Nash Court
John Smith Drive
Oxford Business Park
Oxford
OX4 2RT
Tel: 01865 714455
Fax: 01865 782231
Website: www.potato.org.uk

British Society for Rheumatology

The British Society for Rheumatology (BSR) is a medical society committed to advancing knowledge and practice in the field of rheumatology. We aim to improve awareness and understanding of arthritis and other musculoskeletal conditions and work at national and local level to promote high quality standards of care for people with these conditions.
41 Eagle Street
London, WC1R 4TL
Tel: 020 7242 3313
Fax: 020 7242 3277
e-mail: bsr@rheumatology.org.uk
Website: www.rheumatology.org.uk

British Sports Trust

The British Sports Trusts goal is simple: to help people discover their potential through sport and provide an opportunity to share those abilities with others.
Website: www.bst.org.uk

The British Walking Federation

The British Walking Federation provides many opportunities for people to make friends and enjoy the British countryside through its programme of organised non-competitive events. Its aim is to provide outdoor sports, free from competition, for people of all ages.
BWF National Office
112 Crescent Road
Reading
Berks
RG1 5SW
e-mail: info@bwf-ivv.org.uk
Website: www.bwf-ivv.org.uk

British Wheelchair Sports Foundation

The British Wheelchair Sports Foundation (BWSF) is the national organisation for wheelchair sport in the UK. The Foundation exists to provide, promote and develop opportunities for men, women and children with disabilities to participate in recreational and competitive wheelchair sport.
Stoke Mandeville Stadium
Guttmann Road
Stoke Mandeville
Buckinghamshire
HP21 9PP
Tel: 01296 395995
Fax: 01296 424171
e-mail: info@bwsf.org.uk
Website: www.bwsf.org.uk

British Wheel of Yoga

The British Wheel of Yoga is the largest Yoga organisation in the country and has been registered as a charity for more than 30 years. We are also recognised by the Sports Councils as the national Governing Body for Yoga in the UK.
Central Office
25 Jermyn Street
Sleaford
Lincolnshire
NG34 7RU
Tel: 01529 306 851
Fax: 01529 303 233
e-mail: information@bwy.org.uk
Website: bwy.org.uk/

The British Wrestling Association (BWA)

The BWA website which provides information on wrestling in Great Britain (England, Northern Ireland, Scotland and Wales).
12 Westwood Lane
Brimington
Chesterfield, S43 1PA
Tel/Fax: 01246 236443
e-mail: admin@britishwrestling.org
Website: www.britishwrestling.org

Cardiomyopathy Association

The Cardiomyopathy Association is a registered charity which helps sufferers, their families and their medical advisors to best manage the impact of cardiomyopathy.
40 The Metro Centre
Tolpits Lane
Watford
Herts, WD18 9SB
Tel: 01923 249 977 or
0800 018 1024 (freephone)
Fax: 01923 249 987
e-mail: info@cardiomyopathy.org

CCPR

As the independent voice of UK Sport the CCPR is the umbrella organisation for the national governing and representative bodies of sport and recreation in the UK, speaks and acts to promote, protect and develop the interests of sport and physical recreation at all levels.
Francis House
Francis Street
London, SW1P 1DE
Tel: 020 7854 8500
Fax: 020 7854 8501
e-mail: info@ccpr.org.uk
Website: www.ccpr.org.uk

The Central Council of Physical Recreation

The CCPR is the independent voice of UK Sport and is an umbrella organisation for the national governing and representative bodies of sport and recreation throughout the UK.
Francis House
Francis Street
London, SW1P 1DE
Tel: 020 7854 8500
Fax: 020 7854 8501
e-mail info@ccpr.org.uk
Website: www.ccpr.org.uk/

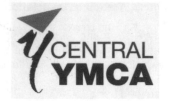

Central YMCA
Central YMCA is the World's founding YMCA, established in 1844 and today internationally renowned for educational programmes within the field of health and fitness.
112 Great Russell St
London, WC1B 3NQ
Tel: 020 7343 1700
e-mail: d.mcintyre@centralymca.org.uk
Websites:
www.ymcaclub.co.uk
www.cyq.org.uk
www.ymcafit.org.uk

Chest, Heart and Stroke Scotland
Chest, Heart and Stroke Scotland aims to improve the quality of life for people in Scotland affected by chest, heart and stroke illness through medical research, advice and information, and support in the community.
Head Office
65 North Castle Street
Edinburgh
EH2 3LT
Tel: 0131 225 6963
Fax: 0131 220 6313
e-mail: admin@chss.org.uk
Head Office: 0131 225 6963
Advice Line: 0845 077 6000
e-mail: adviceline@chss.org.uk
Website: www.chss.org.uk/

The Child Growth Foundation
The Child Growth Foundation is an independent charity and receives no central government or local government funding. It must provide for itself. The Foundation supports children, families of children and adults with growth related problems. It also funds research into possible solutions to these growth related disorders.
2 Mayfield Avenue
Chiswick
London , W4 1PW
Tel: 020 8995 0257
Fax: 020 8995 9075
e-mail: cgflondon@aol.com
Website: childgrowthfoundation.org

The Children's Heart Federation (CHF)
CHF is a federation of local and national support groups. Families in these groups live throughout the UK and Ireland. We provide a freephone helpline and e-mail service, respite care, family support grants, blood test monitors for home use, and a network of computers in hospitals so children can continue their education. We try to raise awareness of the existence and needs of heart children.
Tel: 0808 808 5000
Website: www.childrens-heart-fed.org.uk/

The Chinese National Healthy Living Centre
We aim to promote healthy living, and to provide access to health services, for the Chinese community in the UK. The Centre takes an holistic approach, tackling both the physical and psychological aspects of health.
29-30 Soho Square
London, W1D 3QS
Tel: 020 7534 6546 or 020 7287 0904
Fax: 020 7534 6545
e-mail: general@cnhlc.org.uk
Website: www.cnhlc.org.uk

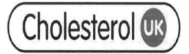

A joint initiative of H•E•A•R•T UK
and the British Cardiac Patients Association

Cholesterol UK
Cholesterol UK is an initiative of two leading heart charities. H•E•A•R•T UK and the British Cardiac Patients' Association. Greater population-wide understanding of heart health risks would help to improve the nation's health and well-being. Cholesterol UK calls for the targeting of raised cholesterol levels, alongside other major risk factors, through education and awareness of diet and lifestyle change.
35 Bedford Row
London, WC1R 4JH
Tel: 0207 400 4480
Fax: 020 7400 4480
e-mail: info@cholesteroluk.org.uk
Website: www.cholesteroluk.org.uk

Colon Cancer Concern
Colon Cancer Concern (CCC) is the UK's leading charity dedicated to reducing deaths from bowel cancer and improving the quality of life of those affected by the disease.
7 Rickett Street
London, SW6 1RU
Tel: 020 7381 9711
Fax: 020 7381 5752
Website: www.coloncancer.org.uk

Consensus Action on Salt and Health (CASH)
CASH (Consensus Action on Salt and Health) is a group of specialists concerned with salt and its effects on health. It is successfully working to reach a consensus with the food industry and Government over the harmful effects of a high salt diet, and bring about a reduction in the amount of salt in processed foods as well as salt added to cooking, and at the table.
Blood Pressure Unit,
Department of Medicine
St George's Hospital Medical School
Cranmer Terrace
London, SW17 0RE
Tel: 020 8725 2409
Fax: 020 8725 2959
Website: www.actiononsalt.org.uk/

CORDA (The Coronary Artery Disease Research Association)
Supports clinical research into the prevention and early diagnosis of cardiovascular disease through the development and application of safe and painless non-invasive methods.
Chelsea Square
London, SW3 6NP
Tel: 020 7349 8686
Fax: 020 7349 9414
Website: www.corda.org.uk

The Coronary Prevention Group (CPG)
The Coronary Prevention Group (CPG) was formed in 1979 by a group of doctors, epidemiologists and other experts in response to the inaction following the 1974 Department of Health Report and the 1976 Report of the Royal College of Physicians and the British Cardiac Society.
e-mail: cpg@lshtm.ac.uk
Website: www.healthnet.org.uk/cpg/

The Counterweight Programme
The Counterweight Programme was launched in 2000 as the result of a national group of consultant physicians recognising the need to tackle obesity management in primary care. The National Counterweight Project Board was established for project guidance and management. Counterweight is a multi-centre practice nurse-led obesity management project being conducted in 80 general practices in 7 regions of the UK.
Westburn House
Foresterhill
Aberdeen
AB25 2ZW
e-mail: hazel.ross@counterweight.org
Website: www.counterweight.org

The Countryside Recreation Network (CRN)
CRN is a network which covers the UK and the Republic of Ireland, gives easy access to information on countryside and related recreation matters, reaches organisations and individuals in the public, private and voluntary sectors, and networks thousands of interested people.
Leisure Industries Research Centre
Sheffield Hallam University
Unit 1, Sheffield Science Park
Howard Street
Sheffield
S1 2LX
Tel: 0114 225 4494
Fax: 0114 225 4488
e-mail: CRN@shu.ac.uk
Website:
www.countrysiderecreation.org.uk

Cricket
Website: www.play-cricket.com

Cycling
www.sustrans.org.uk

Cycling Ireland
Cycling Ireland is the governing body for the sport of cycling in Ireland.
Kelly Roche House
619 North Circular Road
Dublin 1
Ireland
Tel: 01 8551522
Fax: 01 8551771
Website: www.cyclingireland.ie/

Cyclists' Touring Club (CTC)
CTC is the UK and Ireland's largest and longest established national cycling membership organisation. CTC provides a wide range of activities and services designed to enhance the riding opportunities for existing cyclists and make it easier for new entrants to take up cycling.
69 Meadrow
Godalming
Surrey
GU7 3HS
Tel: 0870 873 0060
Fax: 0870 873 0064
e-mail: cycling@ctc.org.uk
Website: www.ctc.org.uk

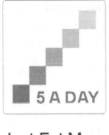

Just Eat More
(fruit & veg)

The Department of Health
The Department of Health's activities to improve diet and nutrition and tackling obesity include reducing the consumption of fat, salt, sugar in the diet, as well as increasing physical activity. The 5 a day programme recommends a variety of a least 5 portions of fruit and vegetables a day.
Website: www.5aday.nhs.uk/

Diabetes Federation of Ireland
Since 1967 the Diabetes Federation of Ireland has been dedicated to helping people with diabetes. Through its network of support branches throughout the country, people who have an interest in diabetes are dedicated to sourcing and sharing information on diabetes and related matters.
76 Lower Gardiner Street
Dublin 1, Ireland
Tel: 01 836 3022
Fax: 01 836 5182
Helpline: 1850 909 909
e-mail: info@diabetes.ie
Website: www.diabetes.ie

Diabetes UK
Diabetes UK is the largest organisation in the UK working for people with diabetes, funding research, campaigning and helping people live with the condition.
Central Office
10 Parkway
London, NW1 7AA
Tel: 020 7424 1000
Careline: 0845 120 2960 (Monday to Friday, 9am to 5pm)
Website: www.diabetes.org.uk

Dieticians working in Obesity Management (UK) [DOM (UK)]
Designed with dieticians in mind, we hope it inspires and informs, and leaves you eager to learn more. Keep a regular lookout for new topical updates, training events, forthcoming meetings, references and resources.
20 Brook Meadon Close
Woodford Green
Essex, IG8 9NR
Tel: 020 8503 2042
e-mail: chris@domuk.ndo.co.uk
Website: www.domuk.org

Diet-i.com
A commercial site with reviews of the various diets.
Website: www.diet-i.com

Different Strokes
Different Strokes is a registered charity providing a unique, free service to younger stroke survivors throughout the United Kingdom. Our services and the number of stroke survivors benefiting from them have grown dramatically since we were formed in 1996. We are run by stroke survivors for stroke survivors, for active self help and mutual support.
9 Canon Harnett Court
Wolverton Mill
Milton Keynes, MK12 5NF
Tel: 0845 130 71 72
e-mail: info@differentstrokes.co.uk
Website: www.differentstrokes.co.uk/

Digestive Disorders Foundation

The Digestive Disorders Foundation is the only national charity that covers the entire range of digestive disorders.
3 St Andrew's Place
London , NW1 4LB
Tel: 020 7486 0341
e-mail: ddf@digestivedisorders.org.uk
Website: www.digestivedisorders.org.uk

DIPEx Charity

DIPEx is an Oxford based charity which produces a unique, award winning website about people's experiences of health and illness. It aims to give information and support to patients, their family and carers so that they are better informed about the life choices they may need to make.

Interviews and information are displayed on the website through a series of video, audio and written interviews, detailing different aspects of the patients' individual experiences from initial diagnosis through to the symptoms, treatments and side effects of the particular disease or condition. As well as answers to frequently asked questions and reliable medical information there are links to support groups and other useful materials.
7200 The Quorum
Oxford Business Park North
Oxford, OX4 2JZ
Tel: 01865 487176
e-mail: info@dipex.org
Website: www.dipex.org

Disabled Living Foundation (DLF)

The DLF are the leading UK disability charity providing advice and information on equipment for independent living. We provide completely impartial advice and information free to the public through our Advice Services Helpline and Equipment Demonstration Centre (EDC), a comprehensive training programme, IT (Sara Project) and the UK's only equipment database.
380-384 Harrow Road
London , W9 2HU
Tel: 020 7289 6111
Website: www.dlf.org.uk/

Disability Sport England

Disability Sport England is the number one events agency for people with all disabilities. We currently run 12 National Championships and 200 Regional Events in a variety of sports. DSE runs a free membership scheme for clubs/schools, organisations and individuals. We are not Government funded so rely on sposorship and fundraising initiatives.
Website: www.disabilitysport.org.uk

Drinkline

Offers help to callers worried about their own drinking, support to the family and friends of people who are drinking, and advice to callers on where to go for help.
Tel: 0800 917 8282 (freephone)

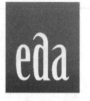

Eating Disorders Association

Eating Disorders Association is a UK wide charity providing information, help and support for anyone affected by or caring for someone affected by an eating disorder, in particular anorexia nervosa, bulimia nervosa and binge eating disorder.
103 Prince of Wales Road
Norwich, NR1 1DW
Adult helpline: 0845 634 1414 (Monday to Friday, 8.30am to 8.30pm; Saturday, 1pm to 4.30pm)
Youthline: 0845 634 7650 (Monday to Friday, 4pm to 6.30pm; Saturday, 1pm to 4.30pm)
Website: www.edauk.com

English Amateur DanceSport Association

The EADA is the governing body for, and the voice of, Amateur Competitive Dancesport in England. As well as being a member of the International Dancesport Federation (IDSF), EADA is the only UK Dancesport Association (Professional or Amateur) which is recognised and supported by Sport England.
Four Winds
Old Potbridge Road
Winchfield, Hampshire, RG27 8BT
Tel/Fax: 01252 843501
e-mail: webmaster@eada.org.uk
Website: www.eada.org.uk

England Basketball

England Basketball aims to create and increase access to sustainable, affordable and regular participation in Basketball. To develop a structure which will enable all players to achieve their full potential in basketball.
c/o English Institute of Sport
Coleridge Road
Sheffield, S9 5DA
Tel: 0870 77 44 225
Fax: 0870 77 44 226
Website: www.englandbasketball.co.uk/

England Squash

England Squash is responsible for the organisation and promotion of squash in England. It is a company limited by guarantee and comprises 38 County Associations, approximately 1,000 Clubs (who affiliate to the organisation on behalf of their members) and Individual and Player members.
National Squash Centre
Sportcity
Manchester, M11 3FF
Website: www.englandsquash.com

English Federation Of Disability Sport

English Federation Of Disability Sport is the Governing Body for Disability Sport in England, as well as the national body responsible for developing sport for disabled people in England.
Manchester Metropolitan University
Alsager Campus, Hassall Road
Alsager, Stoke on Trent, ST7 2HL
Tel: 0161 247 5294
Fax: 0161 247 6895
Minicom: 0161 247 5644
e-mail federation@efds.co.uk

English Karate

English Karate sets the nationally recognised standards and definitions in all aspects of karate in England and this encompasses such vital areas as: Coaching, tournament, club structure, standards of safety, and the protection of children and vulnerable people.
23 Sidlaws Road, Cove
Farnborough, Hants, GU14 9JL
e-mail: info@ekgb.org.uk
Website: www.ekgb.org.uk

English Sports Association For People With A Learning Disability

Works with people with moderate learning difficulties. People with mild and moderate learning difficulties are excluded from society because their strengths are not valued and their needs are not recognised. Their aim is to identify and promote the best ways of

supporting people to live their lives in the way they want to.
ESAPLD
Unit 9, Milner Way, Ossett
West Yorkshire, WF5 9JN
Tel: 08451 298992
Fax: 01924 267 666
email: info@esapld.co.uk
Website: www.esapld.co.uk

The English Volleyball Association

This is the Official Site for Volleyball in England, and carries information regarding all Volleyball Events, News from around the Country and Links to approved English Volleyball Websites and International Sites.
Tel: 01509 631 699. Fax: 01509 631 689
e-mail: general@eng-volleyball.demon.co.uk
Website: www.volleyballengland.org

Everyman

Everyman was established by The Institute of Cancer Research to raise awareness and fund vital research for prostate and testicular cancer. Money raised goes to support the UK's first centre dedicated to male cancers – their diagnosis, prevention and treatment.
The Institute of Cancer Research
Freepost LON 922
London, SW7 3YY
Tel: 0800 731 9468. Fax: 020 7970 6018
e-mail: everyman@icr.ac.uk
Website: www.icr.ac.uk/everyman/

Fencing

Website: www.britishfencing.com

Field sports

Website: www.ukathletics.org

Fighting Fit

Fighting Fit is Manchester Learning Disability Partnership's strategy to encourage and support individuals to lead physically active lifestyles, to eat healthy food, and to achieve or maintain a healthy weight.
MLDP
Mauldeth House, Mauldeth Road West
Chorlton, Manchester, M21 7RL
Tel: 0161 958 4014
Website:
www.mldp.org.uk/fighting%20fit.html

Fitness Industry Association

The Fitness Industry Association (FIA) is the trade body for the health and fitness sector with over 1600 operator members including all the major chain operators and in excess of 100 suppliers.
4th Floor, 61 Southwark Street
London, SE1 0HL
Tel: 020 7202 4700
Fax: 020 7202 4701
e-mail: info@fia.org.uk
Website: www.fia.org.uk

Focus on Food Campaign

The Focus on Food Campaign is an RSA (Royal Society for the encouragement of Arts, Manufacturers and Commerce) flagship education initiative. The Campaign aims to raise the profile and importance of practical food education and help secure, sustain and strengthen the position and status of food in the National Curriculum.
Dean Clough
Halifax, HX6 4LU
01422 383 191
e-mail: helen@design-dimension.co.uk
Website:
www.waitrose.com/focusonfood

The Food Commission

Good food should be tasty, nutritious and safe to eat – so why is our food a major cause of preventable diseases such as obesity, cancer and strokes? The Food Commission is an independent, not-for-profit organisation which investigates these issues and campaigns for safer, healthier food in the UK.
94 White Lion Street
London, N1 9PF
Tel: 020 7837 2250
Fax: 020 7837 1141
Website: www.foodcomm.org.uk

Food Finder

Lists the nutrition information of meals served in popular fast food chains. Use it to find the healthiest item on the menu.
Website: www.olen.com/food

Foodfitness

Food & Drinks Federation's foodfitness programme is a healthy lifestyle initiative with a unique dual approach: promoting enjoyable, healthy eating combined with increased moderate physical activity.
c/o Food and Drink Federation
6 Catherine Street
London, WC2B 5JJ
Tel: 020 7836 2460
Fax: 020 7379 0481
e-mail: foodfitness@fdf.org.uk
Website: www.foodfitness.org.uk

Food Poverty Projects Database

The Food Poverty Projects database (formerly called the Food and Low Income Database) provides an invaluable indication of community food projects across the UK, which tackle food poverty at a community level.
Food Poverty Team
Sustain: The Alliance for Better Food and Farming
94 White Lion Street
London, N1 9PF
Tel: 020 7837 1228, Fax: 020 7837 1141
e-mail: Sustain@sustainweb.org
Website: www.nhsinherts.nhs.uk/hp/health_topics/nutrition/food_poverty_projects_database.htm

Food Standards Agency

The Food Standards Agency is an independent food safety watchdog set up by an Act of Parliament in 2000 to protect the public's health and consumer interests in relation to food.
Aviation House
125 Kingsway
London, WC2B 6NH
Tel: 020 7276 8000
Website: www.food.gov.uk or www.eatwell.gov.uk/

Food for Thought

Oxford Brookes University site aimed at students, but contains important healthy eating tips for anyone on a low income.
Website:
cs3.brookes.ac.uk/student/services/health/food

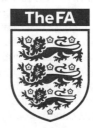

The Football Association

The Football Association is the governing body for football in England, and seeks to develop the sport at all levels under the vision of 'using the power of football to build a better future'.
25 Soho Square, London, W1D 4FA
Tel: 020 7745 4599
e-mail: Health@TheFA.com
Website: www.TheFA.com

Football Foundation

The Football Foundation is the UK's largest sports charity with a £53m per year investment into our communities. By improving the state of our national game and investing in the health of our country we will harness the power of the game to be a force for good in society.
25 Soho Square
London, W1D 4FF
Helpline: 0800 0277766
Tel: 020 7534 4210
Fax: 020 7287 0459
e-mail: enquiries@footballfoundation.org.uk
Website: www.footballfoundation.org.uk

go4awalk.com

On the award-winning go4awalk.com you will find over 6,800 pages of information (with over 1450 photographs) about walking Britain's countryside including the best online UK walk route maps and directions available for walking the Lake District, Snowdonia, the Yorkshire Dales and the Brecon Beacons.
c/o TMDH Limited
PO Box 323
Altrincham, WA14 6YF
e-mail: help@go4awalk.com
Website: www.go4awalk.com

Golf

Website: www.englishgolfunion.org

Great Britain Wheelchair Basketball Association

The objects for which The Association is established are to relieve those persons who have a severe permanent physical disability of one or both lower extremities who are resident in Great Britain or eligible to play for Great Britain by encouraging and promoting the sport of wheelchair basketball with the object of improving conditions of life and to assist in their integration into society.
GBWBA Office
Suite B
Technology Centre
Epinal Way
Loughborough
Leicestershire, LE11 3GE
Tel: 01509 631671
Fax: 01509 631672
Mobile: 07748 668395
e-mail: c.bethel@gbwba.org.uk
Website: www.gbwba.org.uk

Green Gym

BTCV Green Gym offers people an alternative – the opportunity to improve their fitness by involvement in practical conservation activities such as planting hedges, creating and maintaining community gardens, or improving footpaths.
BTCV Conservation Centre
163 Balby Road
Doncaster
South Yorkshire
DN4 0RH
Tel: 01302 572 244
Fax: 01302 310 167
e-mail: Information@btcv.org.uk
Website: www.btcv.org/greengym

Healthy Living Scotland

Here you'll find out about healthy eating and physical activity, and how small changes can lead to big benefits.
Website: www.healthyliving.gov.uk

Health of Men Healthy Living Initiative

The present day HOM project is a 5 year Big Lottery Fund initiative which addresses the neglected area of men's health and the inequalities which result from this historic lack of attention across the Bradford and Airedale district.
e-mail: Chris.andrews@bradford.gov.uk
Website: www.healthofmen.com/

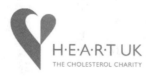

H•E•A•R•T UK

HEART UK is committed to raising awareness of heart disease in the UK and stressing the importance of a healthy lifestyle in reducing the risk of suffering from it.
7 North Road
Maidenhead
Berkshire
SL6 1PE
Tel: 01628 628 638
Fax: 01628 628 698
e-mail: ask@heartuk.org.uk
Website: www.heartuk.org.uk/

HeartLine Association

We are a voluntary organisation set up to offer help and support to children with heart disorders and their families regardless of how slight or severe the condition may be.
Community Link
Surrey Heath House
Knoll Road
Camberley
Surrey
GU15 3HH
Tel: 01276 707636
Fax: 01276 707642
e-mail: admin@heartline.org.uk
Website: www.heartline.org.uk/

Hearts for life

Hearts for life is an interactive educational website to help you understand your heart and its problems.
Website: www.heartsforlife.co.uk/

Heart Throbs4309

Heart Throbs is now one of the leading and most active cardiac support groups in the North London, Middlesex and Hertfordshire
e-mail: info@heart-throbs.org.uk

Help the Aged

Help the Aged is working hard for a world in which older people are valued for their contribution to society, involved in their local communities and fulfilled in their needs, hopes and aspirations.
207-221 Pentonville Road
London
N1 9UZ
Tel: 020 7278 1114
Fax: 020 7278 1116
e-mail: info@helptheaged.org.uk
Website: www.helptheaged.org.uk

High Blood Pressure Foundation

The foundation aims to improve the basic understanding, assessment, treatment and public awareness of high blood pressure and help promote the welfare of people with high blood pressure. The website includes information on the foundation's research, publications and further links.
Director, Rosalind Newton
Department of Medical Sciences
Western General Hospital
Edinburgh
EH4 2XU
Tel: 0131 332 9211
Fax: 0131 537 1012
e-mail: hbpf@hbpf.org.uk
Website: www.hbpf.org.uk

Hoops

Hoops has been online since 1997, offering links and information to the basketball community. Hoops aims to: appeal to all levels of involvement, from those new to the game to those with international experience, to facilitate increased enjoyment, exposure and participation in basketball, to be a source of information, advice and guidance that is relevant, accurate and interesting, to facilitate easier communication within the basketball community.
e-mail: webmaster@hoops.co.uk
Website: www.hoops.co.uk

IBS Network

The mission of the IBS Network is to inform, support, and educate those with IBS and their families and carers; to improve the quality of life of those with IBS and to raise public awareness of IBS and the issues surrounding this condition.
Northern General Hospital
Sheffield, S5 7AU
Tel: 0114 261 1531
Fax: 0114 261 0112

Inclusive Fitness Initiative

The IFI run under the auspices of the English Federation of Disability Sport (EFDS) provides a range of solutions to barriers that make fitness suites inaccessible for disabled people.
04 Park Square
Newton Chambers Road
Thorncliffe Park
Chapeltown
Sheffield, S35 2PH
Tel: 0114 257 2060
Fax: 0114 257 0664
Website: www.inclusivefitness.org/

Institute of Food Research

Information sheets on health issues to do with food, including guidelines for a healthier diet.
Norwich Research Park
Colney
Norwich, NR4 7UA
Tel: 01603 255 000
Fax: 01603 507 723
Website: www.ifrn.bbsrc.ac.uk

The Institute of Leisure and Amenity Management (ILAM)

The Institute of Leisure and Amenity Management (ILAM) is the professional body for the leisure industry and represents the interests of leisure managers across all sectors and specialisms of leisure.
ILAM House
Lower Basildon
Reading, RG8 9NE
Tel: 01491 874800
Fax: 01491 874801
e-mail: info@ilam.co.uk
Website: www.ilam.co.uk

International Association for the Study of Obesity

The IOTF is working to alert the world of the growing health crisis threatened by soaring levels of obesity.
231 North Gower Street
London
NW1 2NS
Tel: 020 7691 1900
Fax: 020 7387 6033
Website: www.iaso.org or www.iotf.org
e-mail: inquiries@iaso.org or obesity@iotf.org
Website: www.iotf.org/

The Irish Heart Foundation

The Irish Heart Foundation is the only national voluntary organisation in Ireland working to reduce premature death and disability from heart disease and stroke through research, education and community service.
4 Clyde Road
Ballsbridge
Dublin 4
Ireland
Tel: 01 6685001
Fax: 01 6685896
Website: www.irishheart.ie

Join the Activaters

Join the Activaters is an interactive education programme for primary school children aged 7-9 (key stage 2). Balancing a healthy diet and being more physically active are increasingly important for young children. Join the Activaters uniquely combines these two elements into one programme.
Foodfitness
c/o Food and Drink Federation
6 Catherine Street
London
WC2B 5JJ
Tel: 020 7836 2460
Fax: 020 739 0481
e-mail: foodfitness@fdf.org.uk
Website: www.jointheactivaters.org.uk

Karate

Website: www.ekgb.org.uk

Keep Fit Association

The Keep Fit Association has keep fit classes running in most parts of the country. There are nine regional organisations. The Keep Fit Association gives people the opportunity to get together in a spirit of fun and friendship to exercise regularly together.
Astra House
Suite 1.05
Arklow Road
London
SE14 6EB
Tel: 020 8692 9566
Fax: 020 8692 8383
e-mail: kfa@keepfit.org.uk
Website: www.keepfit.org.uk/

The Lawn Tennis Association

The Lawn Tennis Association is an organisation bound together by a lifelong passion for the game.
As the governing body of British tennis we are united in our commitment to growing the sport throughout the country at all levels; from the grass roots of the game, to success on the international stage.
Palliser Road
West Kensington
London
W14 9EG
Tel: 020 7381 7000
Fax: 020 7381 5965
Website: www.lta.org.uk

LifeBytes

Site for 11- to 14-year-olds, giving health information in a fun and interesting way. Includes section on healthy eating.
Website: www.lifebytes.gov.uk

Life Cycle UK

Life Cycle UK's vision is of healthy individuals, inclusive communities and an unspoilt natural environment. We work towards these goals by promoting a form of travel that is simple, affordable and equitable – the bicycle!
86 Colston Street
Bristol
BS1 5BB
Tel: 0117 929 0440
Fax: 0117 927 7774
e-mail: post@lifecycleuk.org.uk
Website: www.lifecycleuk.org.uk

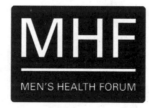

LighterLife

LighterLife is a medically monitored weight loss programme for the obese. Using a nutritionally complete Very Low Calorie Diet in conjunction with Cognitive Behavoural Therapy, clients step back from conventional food to enable them to be in ketosis which blunts hunger, whilst the CBT counselling helps them to explore the reasons behind their overeating.
Tel: 08700 664747
e-mail: inform@lighterlife.co.uk
Website: www.lighterlife.co.uk

Living Streets

The Living Streets initiative is a clear and urgent challenge to the authorities who, for decades, have allowed traffic priorities to overwhelm our local streets and public places, and failed to keep them clean and safe. The Living Streets initiative is a nationwide – ongoing – campaign to win back the streets for everybody.
31-33 Bondway
London
SW8 1SJ
Tel: 020 7820 1010
Fax: 020 7820 8208
e-mail: info@livingstreets.org.uk
Website: www.livingstreets.org.uk

London Cycling Campaign

The London Cycling Campaign is a member organisation that promotes cycling in Greater London by raising awareness of cycling issues, campaigning to improve conditions for cyclists, and providing services for members.
Unit 228
30 Great Guildford Street
London
SE1 0HS
Tel: 020 7928 7220
Fax: 020 7928 2318
Website: www.lcc.org.uk

The Long Distance Walkers Association

The LDWA is an Association of people with the common interest of walking long distances in rural, mountainous or moorland areas. The LDWA furthers the interests of those who enjoy long distance walking in many ways.
e-mail: Secretary@ldwa.org.uk
Website: www.ldwa.org.uk

Malehealth.co.uk

Run by the Men's Health Forum, malehealth offers fast, free independent information for the man in the street. It's the best starting point for men whatever the health query and includes up to date sections on weight problems, diet and related issues.
Website: www.malehealth.co.uk

Mary Hart Centre for Eating Disorders

The Centre for Eating Disorders – Scotland, is a long established, independent, psychotherapy practice concentrating on helping sufferers of Anorexia, Bulimia and Binge Eating Disorder.
3 Sciennes Road
Edinburgh
EH9 1LE
Tel: 0131 668 3051
Website: www.maryhart.co.uk

Men's Health Forum

Tel: 020 7388 4449
Website: www.menshealthforum.org.uk

Milk For Schools

Milk For Schools is a registered charity in England and Wales, charity registration number 1064361, which was founded in 1994. Our charitable mission statement is to educate the public in the field of school based nutrition.
PO Box 412
Stafford
Staffordshire
ST17 9TF
Tel: 01785 248 345
Fax: 01785 248 345
e-mail: info@milkforschools.org.uk
Website: www.milkforschools.org.uk

Mountain Biking

Website: www.bcf.uk.com

Move4Health

Move4Health campaigns and lobbies to make the physical, cultural, political and social environment more conducive for people being active. It also publicises how activity can promote health and wellbeing, contribute towards tackling the burden of psychological and physical disease to help reduce health inequalities in the UK.
Website: www.move4health.org.uk/

The Muslim Health Network

The Muslim Health Network has been established to play a principle role in promoting, preserving, and protecting health and health education amongst Muslim Communities in the UK.
65a Grosvenor Road
London
W7 1HR
Tel: 020 8799 4475
Fax: 020 8799 4465
e-mail: info@muslimhealthnetwork.org
Website: www.muslimhealthnetwork.org

National Centre for Eating Disorders

54 New Road
Esher
Surrey, KT10 9NU
Tel: 01372 469493

National Heart Forum

The National Heart Forum (NHF) is a leading alliance of over 40 national organisations working to reduce the risk of coronary heart disease in the UK.
Tavistock House South
Tavistock Square
London WC1H 9LG
Tel: 020 7383 7638
Fax: 020 7387 2799
e-mail webenquiry@heartforum.org.uk
Website: www.heartforum.org.uk/

National Heart Research Fund

Research into heart disease and prevention and cures of such complaints with dissemination of results. Provision of help and rehabilitation for those with heart disease.
Concord House, Park Lane
Leeds, LS3 1EQ
Tel: 0113 234 7474
Fax: 0113 297 6208
Website www.heartresearch.org.uk

National Institute for Clinical Excellence (NICE)
Website: www.nice.org.uk

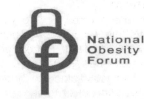

National Obesity Forum
The National Obesity Forum was established in May 2000 to raise awareness of the growing impact of obesity and overweight on our patients and our National Health Service. Membership is open to all healthcare professionals and is free. Through our activities we aim to improve the delivery of best practice in the management of obesity and its co-morbidities. We aim to use all available resources in the media, politically, educationally and professionally to enable all practitioners to confidently treat overweight patients.
National Obesity Forum
PO Box 6625
Nottingham, NG2 5PA
Tel/Fax: 0115 8462109
e-mail: national_obesity.forum@ntlworld.com
Website: www.nationalobesityforum.org.uk/

National Osteoporosis Society
The National Osteoporosis Society (NOS) has is the only national charity dedicated to improving the diagnosis, prevention and treatment of this fragile bone disease.
Camerton
Bath, BA2 0PJ
Tel: 0845 4500230
Fax: 01761 471771
email: nurses@nos.org.uk
Website: www.nos.org.uk/default.asp

The National Playing Fields Association
Protecting and improving playing fields is the core work of The National Playing Fields Association.
Stanley House
St Chad's Place
London, WC1X 9HH
Tel: 020 7833 5360
Fax: 020 7833 5365
e-mail: info@npfa.org
Website: www.npfa.co.uk

NHS Direct
Nurse-led telephone advice and information service. Their website provides a wealth of information and countless links to other resources.
Tel: 0845 4647 24 (24 hour service)
Website: www.nhsdirect.nhs.uk

NHS Smoking Helpline
England and Wales: 0800 169 0169
Scotland and N. Ireland: 0800 848 484
Information in:
Bengali: 0800 169 0885
Gujarati: 0800 169 0884
Hindi: 0800 169 0883
Punjabi: 0800 169 0882
Urdu: 0800 169 0882

The Northern Ireland Chest Heart and Stroke Association
The aim of the Northern Ireland Chest Heart and Stroke Association is to promote the prevention of and alleviate the suffering resulting from chest, heart and stroke related illnesses.
22 Gt Victoria Street
Belfast, BT2 7LX
Tel: 028 9032 0184
Fax: 028 9033 3487
Helpline: 084 5769 7299
Website: www.nichsa.com

The Nutrition Society
The Nutrition Society's aim is to advance the scientific study of nutrition and its application to the maintenance of human and animal health.
10 Cambridge Court
210 Shepherds Bush Road
London
W6 7NJ
e-mail: office@nutsoc.org.uk
Tel: 020 7602 0228
Fax: 020 7602 1756
Website: www.nutritionsociety.org/

Outdoor Industries Association
The Outdoor Industries Association is the lead trade body for manufacturers and retailers of outdoor clothing and equipment.
Morritt House
58 Station Approach
South Ruislip
Ruislip, HA4 6SA
Tel: 020 8842 1111
Fax: 020 8842 0090
e-mail: info@go-outdoors.org.uk
Website: www.go-outdoors.org.uk

The Outward Bound Trust
The Outward Bound Trust is an educational charity that inspires young people to fulfil their potential through challenging outdoor experiences, raising self-esteem and preparing them to face the future. The Outward Bound experience is one which has changed over a million people's lives forever.
Hackthorpe Hall
Hackthorpe
Penrith
Cumbria CA10 2HX
Tel: 08705134227
e-mail: enquiries@outwardbound-uk.org
Website: www.outwardbound-uk.org/

Overeaters Anonymous
PO Box 19
Stretford
Manchester
M32 9EB
Tel: 07000 784985
Website: www.oagb.org.uk

Paths to Health
The Paths to Health Project exists to support the development of local Paths to Health Schemes in Scotland to promote walking for health.
Inglewood House
Tullibody Road
Alloa
FK10 2HU
Tel: 01259 218855
Fax: 01259 218488
e-mail: website@pathsforall.org.uk
Website: www.pathstohealth.org.uk/

Patients' Association
Represents the views and interests of patients to government, health professionals, managers and industry, and campaigns for improved health services. Patient-line providing advice, fact sheets and self-help guides.
PO Box 935
Harrow
Middlesex
HA1 3YJ
Tel: 020 8423 8999
Admin: 020 8423 9111
Fax: 020 8423 9119

The Physical Education Association of the United Kingdom
The Physical Education Association of the United Kingdom is the lead body for physical education in the United

Kingdom, representing the views and interests of nearly 4,000 members of which 3,000 are serving teachers.
Ling House, Building 25
London Road
Reading
RG1 5AQ
Tel: 0118 931 6240
Fax: 0118 931 6242
Website: www.pea.uk.com

The Pituitary Foundation

The Pituitary Foundation is a national UK charity which is working to provide information and support to those suffering from pituitary disorders, their relatives, friends and carers.
PO Box 1944
Bristol
BS99 2UB
e-mail: helpline@pituitary.org.uk
Website: www.pituitary.org.uk

Play-Cricket

Play-Cricket is the ECB's on-line cricket network for all Clubs, Leagues, Cup Competitions and County Boards. It is the official source of all information and statistics on club cricket for all cricketers and supporters.
Tel: 020 7432 1172
Website: www.play-cricket.com

Primary Care Cardiovascular Society

Aims to prevent cardiovascular disease (CVD) and improve care of CVD patients by promoting research, education, and scientific exchange in community-based medicine.
36 Berrymede Road
London
W4 5JD
Tel: 020 8994 8775
Fax: 020 8742 2130
Website: www.pccs.org.uk

The Pulmonary Hypertension Association (UK)

The Pulmonary Hypertension Association (UK) aims to provide support, understanding, and information for all those people whose lives are touched by Pulmonary Hypertension. By bringing people together, and providing a focus for everyone throughout the UK and around the world, the Association aims to make the lives of patients, relatives and carers easier, and more to cope with the challenges that

Pulmonary Hypertension imposes.
PO Box 2760
Lewes
Sussex, BN8 4WA
Tel: 0800 3898 156
Fax: 0701 071 5723
e-mail: enquiries@pha-uk.com
Website: www.pha-uk.com

QUIT

QUIT aims to significantly reduce unnecessary suffering and death from smoking related diseases, and aim towards a smoke free UK future. To provide practical help, advice and support to all smokers who want to stop.
Ground Floor
211 Old Street
London, EC1V 9NR
Tel: 020 7251 1551
Fax: 020 7251 1661
e-mail: info@quit.org.uk
Website: www.quit.org.uk/

Racquetball

Website: www.racquetworld.com

The Ramblers' Association

The Ramblers' Association encourages walking, protects rights of way and defends the beauty of the British countryside. This site provides advice and information about walking in Britain, including: maps and navigation, clothing, equipment and safety, long distance paths, urban walks, walking holidays, walkers and the law.
2nd Floor Camelford House
7-90 Albert Embankment
London, SE1 7TW, UK
Tel: 020 7339 8500
Fax: 020 7339 8501
e-mail:
ramblers@london.ramblers.org.uk
Website: www.ramblers.org.uk

Raising Kids

Site contains healthy eating information for babies, toddlers, young children and teenagers.
Website: www.raisingkids.co.uk

Rowing

Website: www.ara-rowing.org

Rugby Football League

The Rugby Football League (RFL) is the governing body for the game of Rugby League in the UK. It is responsible for all

aspects of the game from promotion and marketing to coaching and national development programs.
Red Hall
Red Hall Lane
Leeds, LS17 8NB
Tel: 0113 232 9111
Fax: 0113 232 3666
e-mail: enquiries@rfl.uk.com
Website: www.rfl.uk.com

Salt Campaign – The Food Standards Agency

This site has been created by the Food Standards Agency to support its salt campaign. The aim of the campaign is to save lives, by reducing the amount of salt people eat. Too much salt can raise your blood pressure, which increases your chances of developing heart disease and stroke.
e-mail: info@salt.gov.uk
Website: www.salt.gov.uk

Scottish Disability Sport

Scottish Disability Sport (formerly the Scottish Sports Association for Disabled People (SSAD)) was formed in 1962 to provide facilities for, and to encourage the development of sport and physical recreation for, disabled people. Scottish Disability Sport has now acted as the governing and co-ordinating body of all sports for all people with a disability for over thirty years.
Caledonia House
South Gyle
Edinburgh, EH12 9DQ
Tel: 0131 317 1130
Fax: 0131 317 1075
e-mail: ssadsds2@aol.com
Website: www.scottishdisabilitysport.com/contactus.cfm

The Scottish Nutrition and Diet Resources Initiative (SNDRi)

The SNDRi aims to produce a range of easily accessible resources on nutrition and diet, which give consistent health messages to the public, and avoid duplication of effort by professionals in Scotland.
Room MS 010 (Milton Street Building)
Glasgow Caledonian University
Cowcaddens Road
Glasgow, G4 0BA
Tel: 0141 331 8481/8479
Fax: 0141 331 8795
e-mail: sndri@gcal.ac.uk

SHARP (Scottish Heart and Arterial disease Risk Prevention)

Aims to reduce the incidence of coronary heart disease in Scotland, mainly through education. Focuses on clinical and scientific meetings and many small local meetings at venues around Scotland.
Ninewells Hospital
Dundee, DD1 9SY
Tel: 01382 660 111
Fax: 01382 660 675
Website www.dundee.ac.uk/sharp

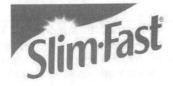

Slim Fast

Slim Fast has been the world's most popular meal replacement weight loss programme for more than 15 years. Its simple structured programme of nutritious meal replacements, satisfying main meals and snacks has been proven to help people lose weight and maintain that weight loss for years.
Tel: 0845 6001311
e-mail:
slimfast@unileverconsumerlink.co.uk
Website: www.slimfast.co.uk

SnowsportGB

The British Ski & Snowboard Federation, trading as Snowsport GB, is made up of 9 constituent member groups, including the Home Nation Governing Bodies plus a number of other organisations who collectively manage British snowsports from grass roots to elite competitive level.
Hillend, Biggar Road
Edinburgh, EH10 7EF
Tel: 0131 445 7676
Fax: 0131 445 4949
e-mail: info@snowsportgb.com

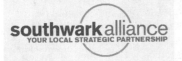

Southwark PCT and Southwark Council

The Southwark Men's Health Programme provides nurse-led outreach MOTs; referral to indoor activities, such as self-defence, swimming and kick boxing; outdoor pursuits such as gardening, accompanied walks, tennis and organised sports; healthy eating advice, cooking and weight management; confidence building workshops and anger management; and personalised smoking cessation and lifestyle programmes.
e-mail: mens.health@southwarkpct.nhs.uk
Website:
www.southwarkpct.nhs.uk/menshealth

Sport England

Sport England is an organisation committed to creating opportunities for people to start in sport, stay in sport and succeed in sport. We provide the strategic lead for sport in England and we are responsible for delivering the Government's sporting objectives. We believe sport has the power to change people's lives.
16 Upper Woburn Place
London, WC1H 0QP
Tel: 020 7273 1613
Fax: 020 7273 1852
e-mail: info@sportengland.org
Website: www.sportengland.org

Sport Scotland

Sport Scotland are committed to putting in place a long-term, sustainable infrastructure for Scottish sport in order to encourage more people to participating in sport.
Caledonia House
South Gyle
Edinburgh, EH12 9DQ
Tel: 0131 317 7200
Fax: 0131 317 7202
e-mail: library@sportscotland.org.uk
Website: www.sportscotland.org.uk/

Sports Council for Northern Ireland

The Sports Council for Northern Ireland aims to make sport happen for the people of Northern Ireland.
House of Sport
Upper Malone Road
Belfast, BT9 5LA
Tel: 028 90 381222
Fax: 028 90 682757
e-mail: info@sportni.net
Website: www.sportni.org/

Sports Council for Wales

The Sports Council for Wales is the national organisation responsible for developing and promoting sport and recreation.
Sophia Gardens
Cardiff, CF11 9SW
Tel: 029 2030 0500
Fax: 029 2030 0600
e-mail: publicity@scw.co.uk
Website: www.sports-council-wales.co.uk/index2.cfm

The Sports Industries Federation

The Sports Industries Federation is the national trade body representing the UK's sporting goods and play industries. With over 20 autonomous trade associations and groups under its umbrella, The Federation covers a wide range of industry sectors including golf, angling, cricket, sports textiles and footwear, play and darts.
6th Street, Avenue E
Federation House, Stoneleigh Park
Warwickshire, CV8 2RF
Tel: 024 7641 4999
Fax: 024 7641 4990
e-mail: admin@sportslife.org.uk
Website: www.thesportslife.com

Sports Leaders UK

Sports Leaders UK believes that everyone has the potential to make a meaningful contribution to their local community – but not everyone has the opportunity or the motivation. Our Sports Leader Awards use the medium of sport to help people learn essential skills such as working with and organising others, as well as motivational, communication and teamwork skills.
Clyde House
10 Milburn Avenue, Oldbrook
Milton Keynes, MK6 2WA
Tel: 01908 689180
Fax: 01908 393744
e-mail: info@sportsleaders.org
Web: Website: www.bst.org.uk

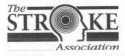

The Stroke Association

The Stroke Association is the only national charity solely concerned with combating stroke in people of all ages. It funds research into prevention, treatment and better methods of

rehabilitation, and helps stroke patients and their families directly through its community services. These include dysphasia support, family support, information services and welfare grants.
240 City Road
London , EC1V 2PR
Tel: 020 7566 0300
Fax: 020 7490 2686
Helpline: 0845 30 33 100
e-mail: info@stroke.org.uk
Website: www.stroke.org.uk

Stroke Survivors
An informational website for victims of stroke, their families, etc.
Website: www.stroke-survivors.co.uk

Sustrans
Sustrans – the sustainable transport charity – works on practical projects to encourage people to walk, cycle and use public transport in order to reduce motor traffic and its adverse effects.
National Cycle Network Centre
2 Cathedral Square
College Green
Bristol , BS1 5DD
Tel: 0117 926 8893
Fax: 0117 929 4173
Website: www.sustrans.org.uk

Table Tennis
Tel: 01494 722525

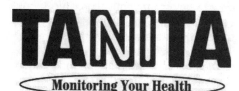

Tanita
Tanita has been a global leader for more than half a century in developing products to help people enjoy a healthier life. Our products are widely used both in the home and professionally by medical and fitness experts.
The Barn
Philpots Close
Yiewsley
Middlesex, UB7 7RY
Tel: 01895 438577
Fax: 01895 438511
Website: www.tanita.co.uk

Tennis
Website: www.tennis.com

thinkvegetables
Thinkvegetables is the definitive source of information about vegetables. The site contains information on how to use and store vegetables, nutritional information for each vegetable and a range of delicious recipes.
c/o M & W Mack Limited
Transfesa Road
Paddock Wood
Kent, TN12 6UT
Tel: 01327 262200
e-mail: info@thinkvegetables.co.uk
Website: www.thinkvegetables.co.uk

The Obesity Awareness & Solutions Trust

TOAST (The Obesity Awareness and Solutions Trust)
TOAST is a national charity (Reg. No. 1088049) dedicated to encouraging a better understanding of obesity, its causes and the practical solutions that are or should be available. We encourage informed debate and research into obesity, and seek to stimulate action for its prevention and treatment. TOAST works closely with industry, academia, patient groups, the medical prefession, consumers, local government and the weight loss industry.
The Latton Bush Centre
Southern Way
Harlow
Essex, CM18 7BL
Tel: 01279 866010
Website: www.toast-uk.org.uk

The Vegetarian Society of the United Kingdom
The Vegetarian Society of the United Kingdom is the oldest vegetarian organisation in the world. It is an educational charity promoting understanding and respect for vegetarian lifestyles.
Parkdale
Dunham Road
Altrincham
Cheshire
WA14 4QG
Tel: 0161 925 2000
Fax: 0161 926 9182
e-mail: info@vegsoc.org
Website: www.vegsoc.org/

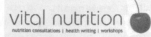

Vital Nutrition
Vital Nutrition is an independent, Belfast based company, offering health workshops for private and corporate clients, one-to-one nutrition consultations for individuals (at Framar Health, Belfast) and health writing for various publications, including local and national newspapers and magazines.
PO Box 430
Belfast, BT8 7YA
Tel: 0775 969 0701
e-mail: info@vital-nutrition.co.uk
Website: www.vital-nutrition.co.uk

Volleyball
Website: www.volleyballengland.org

Walk to School
Site provides the latest news on the national Walking to School initiative. Information for parents, teachers and children. Details of resources and events.
Tel: 020 7820 1010
e-mail: info@livingstreets.org.uk
Website: www.walktoschool.org.uk

Walking Routes
Site provides 700 active lines to web pages containing 1000s of walking-routes, walk descriptions, maps, etc. The directory is organised by county making it easy to find free details of walks in a given area.
Website: www.Walking-Routes.co.uk

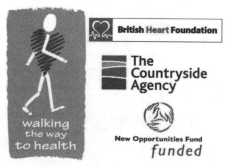

Walking the Way to Health
This WHI website is for everyone with an interest in 'walking for health'. It offers information, support and encouragement

to complete beginners, existing walkers and health and leisure professionals.
The WHI Team
The Countryside Agency
John Dower House
Crescent Place
Cheltenham
GL50 3RA
Tel: 01242 533258
email: jasia.krabbe@countryside.gov.uk
Website: www.whi.org.uk

Water for Health Alliance
Active in promoting drinking water as an essential component of healthcare.
Website: www.waterforhealth.org.uk

Water Polo
Website: www.nwpl.co.uk

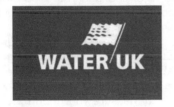

Water UK
Water UK is the industry association that represents all UK water and wastewater service suppliers at national and European level. We actively seek to develop policy and improve understanding in areas that involve the industry, its customers and stakeholders.
1 Queen Anne's Gate
London
SW1H 9BT
Tel: 020 7344 1844
Fax: 020 7344 1866
Website: www.waterforhealth.org.uk

Weight Concern
Weight Concern works to encourage and assist people to control their weight, improve the health and general wellbeing of those who are overweight or obese, provide a reliable source of information on issues relating to obesity, counter prejudice and misinformation, and contribute to the development of more effective obesity treatment programmes.
Brook House
2-16 Torrington Place
London
WC1E 7HN
Tel: 020 7679 6636
Website: www.weightconcern.com

Weight Control Information Network
An American site run by the National Institute of Diabetes and Digestive and Kidney Diseases (NIDDK).
Website: win.niddk.nih.gov/publications/understanding.htm

Weightloss for good
A commercial site with adverts and a sales arm but with useful information and free tools.
Website: www.weightlossforgood.co.uk/

Weightloss resources
A commercial website operating a little like an online group but there are free resources and you can try out the paid-for 'tools' too.
Website: www.weightlossresources.co.uk/

Weight Watchers
For those looking for a group to lose those excess pounds with, Weight Watchers is probably the best known and biggest.
Website: www.weightwatchers.com/international/uk/index.htm

Weightwise
The Weightwise website has been developed, and is managed by, the British Dietetic Association (BDA), the organisation that represents registered dieticians in the UK. The website has been funded by a project grant from the Department of Health and the content written by registered dieticians.
Website: www.bdaweightwise.com

Workplace Health Initiative
Website: www.bhf.org.uk

World Cancer Research Fund (WCRF UK)
Dedicated to saving lives by funding cancer research and providing education programmes that expand our understanding of the importance of our food and lifestyle choices in the cancer process. By spreading the message about cancer prevention through this Website, WCRF UK hopes that countless more lives will be saved.
19 Harley Street
London, W1G 9QJ
Tel: 020 7343 4200
Website: www.wcrf-uk.org/

World Health Organisation
Independent expert report on diet and chronic disease.
Website:
www.who.int/mediacentre/releases/2003/pr20/en/

Wrestling
Website: www.britishwrestling.org

Young TransNet
A project using new technology and the internet to help children and young people walk, cycle and use public transport, and to support parents, schools and local authorities.
National Children's Bureau
Wakley Street
London
EC1V 7QE
Tel: 020 7843 6325
Website: www.youngtransnet.org.uk

Your Overweight Child
Starting point for parents and carers who want to help their overweight child regain confidence and achieve a healthy weight.
Website: www.youroverweightchild.org

The Youth Sport Trust
The Youth Sport Trust is a registered charity established in 1994 by Sir John Beckwith to build a brighter future for young people through sport. Our mission is to support the education and development of all young people through physical education (PE) and sport.
Sir John Beckwith Centre for Sport
Loughborough University
Loughborough
Leicestershire
LE11 3TU
Tel: 01509 226600
Fax: 01509 210851
Website: www.youthsporttrust.org

How your pharmacist can help you lose the pounds but not the £s.

Your local pharmacist (chemist) is your health care professional in the high street and is perhaps the most accessible part of the health service. No appointments are needed, advice is free, there are no long waiting lists and you can get a large range of goods and services to help you fight the inch (25 millimetre) war.

Your pharmacist will supply:
- Condoms – have more safe sex and burn more calories. 20 minutes of sex burns twice the calories of 20 minutes of mixed doubles tennis.
- Perfume/aftershave – buy some for the wife/girlfriend/partner to increase the likelihood of the above!
- A new toothbrush, floss, mouthwash and sugar free gum – look after your mouth and keep it busy and active so it doesn't miss the full English, Welsh, Scottish or Irish fried breakfasts. Will also increase the likelihood of the above!
- Giving up smoking aids – tobacco and nicotine substitutes – gums, patches, lozenges, micro-tablets, and inhalers to will help you stop raiding the biscuit-tin or hitting the bottle by reducing your cravings for fags (and increasing your desire and performance for the above!).
- Pain-killers for your wife/girlfriend as she is probably developing headaches to *decrease* the likelihood of the above!
- Tape measures and weighing scales – car or lorry mirrors, the opinion of Doris in the transport café, the views of your workmates or trying to use HGV weighbridges will not be good enough

to see if your waistline really is shrinking.
- Sweeteners and sugar substitutes – some things in life (except the unceremonious substitution of Gary Lineker by England manager Graham Taylor in the critical Euro 1992 game against Sweden) can be substituted successfully!

Your pharmacist can also give you free help and advice on:
- Figuring out the figures on food labels – understand how "Low Fat" or "Diet" food doesn't always "do what is says on the can".
- Discussing your prescription and over-the-counter medicines – a few medicines contain lots of sugar, some could cause weight gain as a side effect, and some

may not work as well as they should if you have changed your diet, stopped smoking or started drinking grapefruit or cranberry juice, for example.
- Understanding how losing weight will reduce your chances of getting diabetes, high blood pressure or a heart attack. Some pharmacists will be able to measure your blood pressure or cholesterol level for you, so you can see how your health is improving.

Your pharmacist will not supply:
- Laxatives – if you take these to try to lose weight you will be as full of sh*t as you were before!
- Quack diet pills and potions – there is no such thing as a magic pill or potion, the only weight you will lose will be from your wallet!

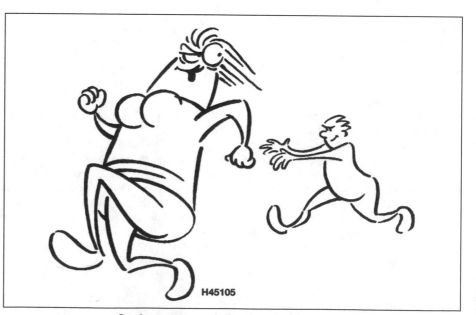

H45105

Sex burns more calories than doubles tennis

Do you see yourself as being on a diet?

It's tempting to see diets as a quick fix – to deny yourself what you like for a short while, then go back to old habits. Instead, think of weight loss as a long-term project, and a change to healthier eating for life. It's better to continue with moderate but effective changes for years, than to try an extreme diet and fail.

Have you set goals?

Setting goals is one of the best ways for you to succeed – this can give you the motivation and direction you need to be successful. See Section 3 in Chapter 6.

Are you clear about *why* you want to lose weight?

What's your motivation for losing weight? Perhaps it is to be fitter, healthier or just plain sexier? Whatever it is, fix this clearly in your mind. Imagine this as vividly as you can. If you like, write it down (or draw a picture) and put it on the wall, or even the fridge. Make definite plans for what you want to do when you achieve your goal.

Have you planned rewards for hitting your targets over coming months?

In the short term, plan rewards for yourself for hitting your targets at 2, 4 and 6 months, etc. Reward yourself with something special for achieving your goals.

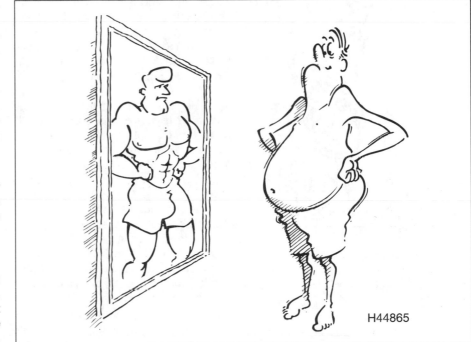

Imagine your intentions as vividly as possible

Are your goals realistic?

It is easy to be overambitious – given the choice we'd all like a body like Brad Pitt, ideally by next week. However change takes time. For example, building up fitness can take many months and is best taken slowly and steadily. A common mistake is to go on an extreme diet to try to lose over 2lbs per week. It is almost always impossible to keep this up. *Weight loss of just 1lb per week is a realistic target, and is probably ideal.*

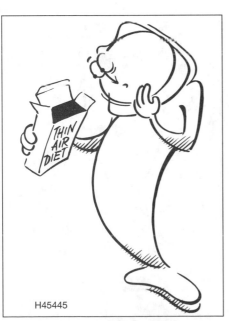

A common mistake is to go on an extreme diet

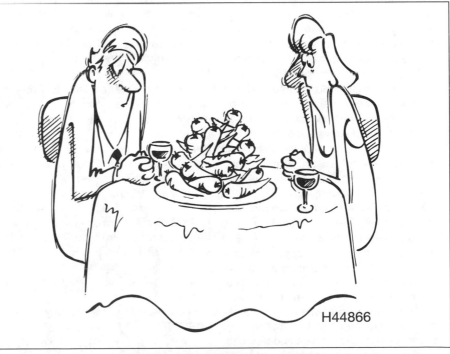

Even the healthiest meals can get boring

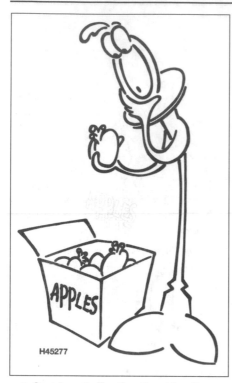

Snack on fruit rather than biscuits

Maintain this rate of weight loss for a year and you will lose nearly 4 stone.

Despite this, are you finding hunger a problem?

Don't skip meals - aim to eat three good meals a day (breakfast, lunch and evening meal). Don't shrink your meals either - eat enough to take you through comfortably to your next meal without hunger. Different approaches suit different people: experiment to find out what type of diet best *satisfies* you. For some, a low-fat diet will work best, for others it will be the Glycaemic Index approach, or a high protein/low carb diet. In all cases, load up on fresh fruit and veg, which are filling, low in calories, and highly nutritious.

Do you find what you're supposed to eat boring, bland or monotonous?

Our taste buds crave new flavours, tastes and experiences; as well as old favourites. If the ingredients you're allowed are restricted (as in some extreme diets) you'll tire of them very quickly. Having only a few recipes to choose from can also soon become very tedious. Get inspiration from cookbooks (any library or bookshop), magazines or even supermarket recipe cards. Invest

some time, and learn some new skills and recipes. Make sure that your diet is varied, with lots of change and interest. Healthy food can not only be simple and quick to make but also incredibly tasty.

Do you have problems finding the time to cook?

Time is short, but what are your priorities? If your diet is making you ill, through overweight or obesity, then you need to take control of it. The only way that you can guarantee the quality of what you eat is to buy with care and cook at home. Like sex, cooking is natural and normal, can be fun and doesn't have to be over in 30 seconds (or last for hours). A reasonable target should perhaps be a maximum of 30 minutes – for cooking and preparation that is. Modern cookery books can help: look for ones that have quick, clear recipes. In some cases you can save time by cooking double quantities, and freezing or refrigerating half to eat later.

Is 'snacking' a problem for you?

If you're snacking because you're hungry, see above. If on occasions you are still hungry then snack on fruit, for example (chocolate biscuits have more than 14 times the calories of an apple or orange). If you're not really hungry, then it may be a habit. Think about where and when you are snacking – what can you do to change this pattern?

Are chocolates, crisps, biscuits, fizzy pops, cakes or fast foods your downfall?

These are all loaded with calories, are heavily advertised and are sold almost everywhere. Start with shopping: just make sure that you don't buy these items (if necessary avoid the aisles or shops containing them). If you don't buy them, you can't eat them. *After all, what is the point of buying food if you are then going to try not to eat it?* These are the highest calorie foods, and simply cutting these out may deliver all the weight loss you need. Use the money that you save to buy good quality ingredients for cooking: fresh fruit & veg, meat, fish, olive oil, etc.

Do you need to cut back on your drinking?

Alcohol is high in calories – for example a pint of beer contains 180 calories. A reduction in intake of 2 to 3 pints per day

represents 3350 calories over a week, which is equivalent to 1lb of weight loss per week. See 'Alcohol and losing weight' (Chapter 6) for more information.

Do you need to exercise more?

Weight is a balance between calorie intake and energy expenditure. The more active you are, the more freedom you can have with your diet.

Do you need to see a doctor?

Sometimes weight gain can be caused by illness, such as an underactive thyroid. Typically, people with this would also feel exceptionally tired. Depression can also cause weight gain in some cases – suspect this if you have become generally low in your spirits, excessively anxious, or if your sleep has become poor. If necessary, your doctor can advise you further. If you are overweight you might want to get your blood pressure checked anyway, and have tests to rule out high cholesterol and diabetes.

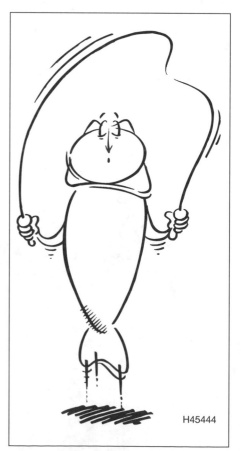

Weight is a balance between calorie intake and energy expenditure

How to lose weight without getting hungry

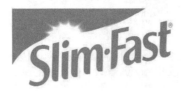

By Dr. Anthony R. Leeds
Data drawn from McCance and Widdowson's The Composition of Foods, 5th Edition, 1991, Cambridge: Royal Society of Chemistry.

When you think of diets you think of counting calories and getting hungry and being miserable. Well does this really have to be the only way to a less-fat you?

The answer is no. Nature and the food technologist together offer you a way out of this dilemma, and all you have to do is exploit what is already there.

To lose weight without specifically trying you'd have to eat foods that make you feel more full, and contain less dietary energy (calories) than the foods you ate before. So you need to use the natural variation on the 'energy density' of foods and the 'filling' nature of foods. Some doctors and dieticians believe, correctly, that you have to start to think about the amounts of food you're eating – and that is absolutely true. You do have to become a 'restrained' (controlled) eater as well. As in every other aspect of life on this planet a degree of restraint is necessary in order to have a tolerable existence alongside everyone else – and diet is no exception. Restraint IS necessary. So you do have to resist that second helping, choose the smaller option, learn polite ways to reject mother-in-law's generous offer of a third helping of her delicious casseroles, chicken tikka massala and sponge pudding, and even deliberately go against basic nature and leave something on the plate.

Oh, and don't eat in front of the television, don't go shopping while you're hungry, and find out what 'triggers' your desire to eat (keep written notes and try to think of ways of avoiding these).

Energy density

Energy density is a measure of how much energy is in a given weight of food. One teaspoon of sugar (about 5g) contains 20 calories – the energy density is 4 calories per gram. At the other extreme a salad vegetable such as lettuce is mostly water. The weight of lettuce that provides 20 calories is 100g (about 20 times as much as would be consumed in one portion) and the energy density is about one fifth of a calorie per gram. Sugar is 20 times more energy dense than lettuce. In between are a variety of other energy densities. If you are trying to lose weight go for the lower energy density foods.

Energy Densities – energy (calories) per 100g of food

Apple	47
Bacon, lean fried	332
Banana	95
Beef, roast	284
Bread, white	235
Bread, wholemeal	215
Cheese, hard, eg, cheddar	405
Chips, fried in oil	239
Choc ice	277
Clotted cream	586
Custard (skimmed milk)	79
Digestive biscuits, plain	471
Fish fingers, grilled	214
Fruit cocktail, canned	57
Haddock, steamed	98
Low fat yoghurt	41
Milk semi-skimmed	46
Milk, whole	66
Omelette, plain	191
Oranges, flesh only	37
Pears	40
Pizza, cheese and tomato	235
Plums	36
Rice pudding, canned	89
Risotto, plain	224
Roast chicken (meat only)	148
Single cream	198
Teacakes, toasted	329
Yorkshire pudding	208

It'll fill you up

You've heard it before: "If you eat porridge for breakfast you won't want to eat anything 'til lunch-time", and actually it's true. The sticky stuff in oat porridge is the dietary fibre which is 'glue-like' in consistency and it really does 'stick-up' your guts so that your stomach empties more slowly, the starch and sugars in the porridge are digested slowly – and you really will feel full for longer.

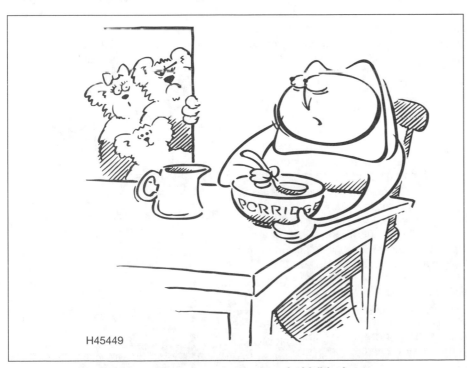

H45449

Porridge sticks-up your guts so you feel full for longer

Eat yourself thin

Are there any other foods that make you feel full for longer? Yes, in fact any food which has a high amount of dietary fibre, but especially soluble fibre (oats, beans and cereal foods like some wholewheat breakfast cereals and some breads, such as granary multi-grain breads) will help you to fill up.

Glycaemic Index and Glycaemic Load

Glycaemic Index (GI) and Glycaemic Load (GL) are the buzz-words of the twenty-first century. GI tells us about how much the blood glucose rises when a carbohydrate food is eaten and GL tells about how much of that GI carbohydrate is in the portion or meal containing the food. There is lots of information about the GI and GL and it's well worth getting to know more about it. But is it true? Do Low GI and Low GL really help people lose weight? Well there is some good evidence and it's slowly building up, but there is another important point about GI: GI only tells us one thing about the food (its GI), but generally Low GI foods have a whole set of very desirable features which help people lose weight. Generally, but not always, Low GI foods are high in dietary fibre, low in energy density and are slowly digested in the gut. The transfer of energy (sugars, fats and proteins) into the blood is slower and you will get stronger messages from your gut to your brain telling you not to eat. It's worth a try – go for Low GI and even give Low GL a try as well.

Protein

Twenty years ago scientists showed that protein foods had a slightly stronger effect on the feeling of hunger than carbohydrate and fat, so for example having a chicken piece with salad for lunch is the way to get through the afternoon and keep the calories down, but not if it's been cooked in fat and is eaten with fat-soaked chips. It'll fill you up but you'll have tucked away another ounce of fat under your belt. So the answer is you can make food choices which mean you use the effect of protein, but it's a waste of time if you do not also watch the total calorie content of the meal.

Can I eat meat? Yes, but GRILL and TRIM!

We've all been taught that meat is full of fat and that you have to cut it down if you're going to reduce that waistline. Well, in response to the concern with fat and heart disease the meat industry (breeders, farmers and butchers) now produce meat cuts with much less fat in them. Lean meat is readily available. So you don't have to miss out on your favourite steak, but make sure it's a really lean cut and is not soaked in fat while it's cooked (grilled rather than fried). If there is any visible fat, you can always trim it off and leave it on the plate. The energy content of lean meats is affected by frying compared to grilling:

Energy content calories per 100g

	Fried	Grilled
Bacon (with lean and fat)	465	405
Lean bacon	332	292
Steak (with lean and fat)	246	218
Lean steak	190	168

That's an impressive reduction in calories while not depriving yourself of a favourite food. The average 8 ounce steak can be 175 calories less if it's lean and grilled rather than a fatty steak fried – that's a big difference for one item on the plate.

So there's nothing new there then?

No, the difference between now and twenty years ago is in knowledge and understanding. We know more about fibre – many high fibre foods are more filling. We now know that energy density is critical to success in controlling body weight – go for the reduced fat and reduced calorie options. The commercial products are now very good, well-designed and tasty. We know about GI and GL – we still need to know more, but in the meantime give Low GI and Low GL a try – they may work for you. We know about the filling effect of protein. Try using lean protein foods as part of a balanced intake over the whole day, but take care if you have diabetes, a history of kidney disease or if your family history suggests that you may develop diabetes. Too much protein in the diet may not be good if you have those problems.

cals and kcals

The terms cal (calorie) and kcal (kilocalorie) are used in the scientific world as measures of energy. kcals are 1000 times larger than cals.

Food is an energy source, so it is useful to be able to quantify the available energy from each portion or 100g.

A lot of foodstuffs are quite energy dense, so their values would tend to run into the tens of thousands. To keep the numbers more manageable, the unit used is the kcal, which is what is printed on the Nutrition Information label on pre-packaged food.

Quite often, foods are described as having a number of calories, but this is just shorthand for kcal not, unfortunately, the real thing.

Nutrition Information		
TYPICAL VALUES	Per ½ Pot	Per 100g As Sold
ENERGY	695kJ (170kcal)	820kJ (200kcal)
PROTEIN	2.7g	3.2g
CARBOHYDRATE of which sugars	6.3g 2.2g	7.4g 2.6g
FAT of which saturates	14.6g 3.5g	17.2g 4.1g
FIBRE	0.1g	0.1g
SODIUM	0.09g	0.10g
SALT EQUIVALENT	0.2g	0.3g
Guideline Daily Amount of Salt for Adults 6g		

Is the food industry pulling its weight?

The food industry? I thought this was a health book. So what's the story?

In the UK, the food we buy is regulated by both EU law and domestic law like the Food Standards Act 1999, but the government is calling on the food industry to do more in the fight against obesity.

So how, er, big is the problem?

In the UK it is estimated that some 20% of men (1 in 5) and 25% of women (1 in 4) are obese. As many as 30,000 people die prematurely every year from obesity-related conditions. The National Audit Office estimates the cost of obesity and related diseases to the NHS as at least £500m a year.

What does the government want the industry to do?

Impose voluntary restrictions on advertising high-fat and high-sugar foods, especially to children. If the government's not satisfied, it says it will impose restrictions by law in 2007. The European Union has made similar threats.

Fat chance. What do the experts say?

The National Obesity Forum (NOF), who are beginning to work with food companies on making their products more healthy, reckon that this 'assisted self-regulation' can work. NOF's David Haslam says the government's strategy is 'pretty shrewd' as it encourages self-regulation but at the same time sets a tight deadline for it.

'The first thing the food industry needs to do is hold its hands up and admit there's a problem,' says David Haslam. 'They do in private, but in public they still say there's no such thing as a bad food only bad diets, they still say obesity is about exercise not diet, they still say they're not trying to attract children with their advertising. None of these things is true.'

Do other countries have regulations on ads?

Yes, food advertising it is already regulated to some degree in Belgium, Denmark, Quebec, Australia, Finland and the Netherlands. In Sweden all advertising aimed at children under 12, all advertising between programmes and all advertising before and after kids' programmes is banned. Their economy has not collapsed.

So do food companies lie in their advertising?

No. But like all of us – businesses, governments, blokes in general – they simply present the information in the way that is best for them.

Take these examples which are mentioned in 'Broadcasting Bad Health', a 2003 report by the International Association of Consumer Food Organizations for the World Health Organization:

- 'Experts continue to agree that for health and enjoyment, we should aim to eat more carbohydrate foods of all kinds, including sugars and starches.' (from British Sugar's Energy for Life education book, 2003)
- 'All soft drinks are healthy because they provide the vital fluids our bodies need.' (from the British Soft Drinks Association's website)

Both of these statements are true but they don't tell the full story. The 'vital fluid' in question is water. 'Carbonated and still drinks are 86% water,' the drinks site says later. True. The question is what's in the other 14%.

But nobody makes you stuff your face, do they?

No. We're all responsible for our own behaviour. In the same way, people selling us food products are responsible for theirs. They need to tell us clearly what's in their food and what these ingredients can do.

David Haslam would like to see far more accurate labelling. 'We are seeing the end of 85% fat-free labels on crisps which is good. That was completely misleading. But it is still no good to call a reduced fat product healthy if it's been bulked up with eight tablespoons of sugar.' He welcomes the Food Standards Agency (www.food.gov.uk) consultation on a signposting system which would show levels of all ingredient types, good and bad.

But is it just about advertising?

No. For David Haslam, who is also a GP, the key issue is actually food content. He's not asking for dramatic changes. 'We need small adjustments, a little at a time. Salt levels have been edging up and up and up. Our taste buds have been numbed. We need to reverse that trend in salt, in sugar, in fats, in additives and in portion sizes.'

Sounds like it could help. What else are campaigners doing?

Criticising food industry profits misses the point. Food companies, like all public companies, are obliged to maximise their profits for their shareholders. That's their job. Campaigners for healthier food are developing a more sophisticated strategy: encouraging the public to demand healthier food.

Is the food industry pulling its weight?

Easier said than done.

True. In Britain, demand for ready-meals grew by 44% between 1990 and 2002. We now consume twice as many ready-meals as the French and six times as many as the Spanish. Longer working hours, rising incomes and increasing numbers of parents out at work mean this pattern is likely to continue.

That sort of food is cheap too.

That's what people think but it's not always true. Supermarkets may be cheaper on 'loss leaders' like milk, baked beans and bread but on many items, especially fresh ones, they're not. Check it out for yourself. Organic fruit and veg from a local shop is often cheaper than pesticide-plastered stuff from the supermarket.

Really?

Campaigners are also pointing out the environmental damage done by food processing and drawing attention to animal cruelty.

OK, so buy organic and free-range produce. But big food companies do a lot for society already. They give computers and other things to schools.

True. It's called CSR.

CSR? Is that a super-bug?

No, it stands for corporate social responsibility and it's very welcome, but not all of those schemes are actually very healthy. One crisp company, for example, gave books to schools in return for tokens from their packets. Even the 'cheapest' book required the child to eat 50 packets of crisps. That weighs in at more than 7,500 calories and over half a kilo of fat.

See what you mean. Can this moral pressure work?

Maybe. That particular crisps campaign is not going anymore and despite their huge size and large profits, many food companies are far more vulnerable to changes in public opinion about their products than you might think. Banks are now warning investors that food companies seen as unhealthy could be putting their share price at risk.

So will the government have to legislate?

Self-regulation works only if the companies concerned want to play ball. The fact is that they have a legal obligation to maximise their profits for their shareholders. Whether legislation is needed or whether the threat of it is sufficient depends how companies interpret this obligation. If they, and their share-holders, take the view that small changes now will be more profitable than larger changes later, there may be no need for new laws.

But have they got the stomach for it?

We'll have to weight and see.

A fuller version of this article was first published on the malehealth web site (www.malehealth.co.uk).

A History of Gluttony

by David Haslam

Think yourself lucky! In the 6th Century, when the Seven Deadly Sins were announced by Pope Gregory the Great, eating too much didn't just lead to an expanding waist line; gluttony lead to eternal damnation in Hell. And to make matters worse, gluttony didn't just mean eating too much or too greedily, it also included eating too early, too delicately, too quickly, and even just having a hearty appetite was enough to end up burning in fire and brimstone for ever.

Lust and gluttony were unique among the Seven Deadly Sins, in that even the most saintly person admitted that sexual intercourse and eating were both necessary for the continuation of the species, so they couldn't be ruled out altogether; the sin was to actually enjoy them. Saint Francis of Assisi added ashes to his food to make sure it was as unpleasant as possible, just so he could be quite free from accusations of gluttony.

What was it about eating too much that was so bad as to be punishable by eternal damnation? And what about Sloth, that other Deadly Sin which also leads to overweight and obesity? The trouble with both transgressions is not what sinners *did,* but what the sins *prevented* them from doing. Eating too much took their minds off holy things, leading to debauchery, drunkenness and temptation, and being slothful merely meant they never got round to doing God's holy work.

Saint Basil complained, rather incoherently, that "The sense of touch in tasting and gluttony by swallowing, the body, fattened up and titillated by the soft humours bubbling uncontrollably inside is carried in a frenzy towards sexual intercourse", and Thomas Aquinas described the six daughters of gluttony: excessive joy, unseemly joy, loutishness, uncleanness, talkativeness and uncomprehending dullness of mind. However, Thomas ended his days being rather soft on gluttony and sloth, maybe because he himself indulged a little, and ended up "looking like a wine barrel", and needing a crescent shape to be cut out from the table to enable him to sit near enough to his food.

The exact fate awaiting gluttons in Hell has been hotly debated among preachers since eternal damnation was announced. The greatest writers and artists have attempted to describe these punishments. Dante suggested that as payment for pandering to the pleasures of the flesh during life, gluttons would be condemned to the third circle of Hell, where they would exist in eternal discomfort, in interminable hail, naked and starving in a swamp. Some said that nourishment would be plentiful: sinners would be surrounded by fine foods and wine, meats, fruit and bread, but that they would be prevented from eating it by demons who would burn them, and impale them on their claws. Others suggested that gluttons would be able to eat and drink as much as they could, but

have a slightly limited menu, being force fed on toads and vermin, and being made to drink fresh urine through a funnel. But the majority seemed to believe that gluttons would themselves be eaten in a variety of different ways: sometimes whole, by demons, sometimes cut into pieces and fried in a pan, or maybe roasted on a spit or boiled in a cauldron.

So in the 6th Century, the advice was the same - avoid overeating and inactivity - but for completely different reasons. Today doctors recommend healthy lifestyles to avoid problems during the rest of our earthly life, rather than in purgatory: problems such as heart disease, diabetes, blood pressure and stroke which are a direct result of excess weight.

However, obesity was known to be a medical problem long before Pope Gregory. Over 3,000 years ago Hippocrates wrote "men who are constitutionally very fat are more likely to die quickly than those who are thin". The differences between the risks of obesity to men as opposed to women were well recognised amongst the Greeks, who realised that obese women were frequently infertile, whereas obese men had a shortened life expectancy. The connection between obesity and respiratory disorders was recognised by Celsus, one of the earliest physicians, who said "The obese are throttled by acute diseases and breathing difficulties; they often die suddenly which rarely happens in the thinner person".

More recently, in the 19th Century, the link between maleness and obesity has been more clearly defined. According to the famed writer and wit Brillat-Savarin "There is one kind of obesity that centres round the belly ... I call this type of fatness Gastrophoria, and its victims Gastrophores. I myself am in their company; but although I carry a fairly prominent stomach, I still have well-formed lower legs, and calves as sinewy as the muscles of an Arabian steed". He is describing the typical (and dangerous) 'apple' shape which obese men tend to assume, as opposed to the 'pear' shape of obese women who often carry their weight harmlessly on the thighs.

Unfortunately it is the 'apples' which have the associated severe risks of obesity related illness. However, one notable 'apple' found the answer to his weight problem: William Banting, who was a coffin maker to the Royal Family in the 1860s. Not only did he succeed in ridding himself of 'this lamentable disease', but he also put pen to paper and wrote the first commercially available diet book, the 'Letter On Corpulence, addressed to the Public'.

Banting's diet is recognised nowadays as the forerunner of the Atkins diet: he cut out bread, sugar, beer and potatoes, and lost over 12 inches off his waist. Unlike modern low-carbohydrate diets, it suggests 7 units of alcohol per day!

In days gone by, swollen waistlines accompanied swollen wallets; only those people who could afford to eat well became fat. If you were choosing a doctor or a lawyer, you would never choose a skinny one! These days the connection between money and weight is not as clear cut. Fast food is cheap and readily available at any time of day and night, but gyms are expensive and exclusive.

Over the entire course of history the most celebrated obese people have been male, and many of them extremely well off. Wealthy Romans would eat vast amounts, then deliberately be sick in a room called a vomitorium, so they could go back for second helpings of hummingbird tongues and goat's testicles. Henry VIII believed that increased girth was a sign of heroic valour, so he deliberately gained weight, until at age 56 his chest measurement was 60 inches, and he could no longer walk around the Palace. Louis XIV of France was not as successful; he resorted to padding his clothes to give him the appearance of obesity. The composer Rossini was immensely proud of his gut, and was known as 'Rossini the Lazy'; if, as he lay in bed composing, he dropped a manuscript, he would rather start a new piece than be bothered to pick it up!

Winston Churchill was another famous 'apple' who spent long hours in bed, eventually controlling the war effort whilst lying there naked. Diamond Jim Brady, the philanthropist, financier and jewel collector, was one of the world's most notorious gluttons. He would allegedly sit down for dinner leaving a gap of 6 inches between his belly and the table, and only rise from dinner once the gap had been filled.

In 1780 Samuel Johnson, the most famous writer and personality of his day, said "Whatever be the quantity that a man eats, it is plain that if he is too fat, he has eaten more than he should have done". His friend James Boswell disagreed, saying "You will see one man fat who eats moderately, and another lean, who eats a great deal". There is a great deal of truth in both statements, and the lesson is that just as there are different causes for becoming apple shaped, so there are different remedies.

Our prehistoric ancestors only survived if they had the ability to store the food they ate as fat, because although one day there might plenty of meat, the next day there might be nothing; times of plenty followed by famine and fast. Cavemen who couldn't lay down fat stores would die as soon as the next famine occurred. In the 21st century, evolution has played a dirty trick. Nowadays those of us who lay down fat stores will die early, and the descendants of those cavemen who got sand kicked in their faces because they were weedy, will survive.

Dieting flies in the face of what our genetic make-up is telling us, which is why it is so difficult. If we buy a fast food burger, deep down we congratulate ourselves for a successful day's hunting; it is extremely difficult, but essential, to override this instinct.

Physical activity is another essential part of attempts to lose weight, but once again, nature has bowled us a googly. Our ancestors looked upon rest as an essential part of life, as they gained adequate exercise from hunting. There were only three reasons for them to leave their cave: to hunt for food, empty their bowels, or have sexual intercourse. Straying from home for any other reason merely increased the risk of becoming dinner for someone or something else. There are no modern diet and exercise plans based on hunting, defecating and having sex, but Dr. Shukan Tokuho of Tokyo has proposed what he calls a masturbation diet:

"The three main advantages of this regimen are that it is quick, easy and good for health. Five minutes of vigorous masturbation can consume 300 calories which is the equivalent of sprinting 100 metres. It can be done while sitting at your desk and the experience is so refreshing that it can replace a light meal, thereby saving more calories. The ideal position is leaning back in a chair with the heels raised about 10 centimetres off the floor, because this puts tension on the stomach muscles. Performed in this way masturbation is as strenuous as doing push-ups or sit-ups in a sauna and can trim 8 centimetres off the waist if performed twice a day for a month, as part of a calorie controlled diet."

The sort of exercise more usually recommended is sport and scheduled activity for those who wish to and are able to, and routine activity built into daily life for everybody. This doesn't mean becoming a lumberjack, merely walking more during the day, using the stairs, walking up escalators and so on.

History is littered with attempts to induce weight loss, often dangerously, often ludicrously, and occasionally successfully. We can learn valuable lessons from our predecessors, but unfortunately as overweight and obesity are now present in the population in epidemic proportions it is vital to find safe and effective remedies, and put them to good use.

Banks, Ian *Ask Dr Ian about Men's Health* (The Blackstaff Press; Belfast, 1997)

Banks, Ian *The Man Manual* (Haynes Publishing; 2002)

Banks, Ian *The Trouble With Men* (BBC; 1997)

Banks, Ian *Get Fit With Brittas* (BBC; 1998)

Banks, Ian *The NHS Direct Healthcare Guide* (Radcliffe Press; 2000)

Baker, Peter *Real Health for Men* (Vega; 2002)

Barrier, Phyllis *Type 2 Diabetes for Beginners* (American Diabetes Association; 2005)

Beck, Carol *Anorexia and Bulimia for Dummies* (Wiley; 2005)

Blakeman, Rob *Passion for a Change: Achieving Real Health in the 21st Century* (Brewin Books; 2005)

Bradford, Nikki *Men's Health Matters: The Complete A-Z of Male Health* (Vermillion; London, 1995)

Brewer, Sarah *The Complete Book of Men's Health* (Which?; London, 1999)

Carpender, Dana *Dana's Carpender's Weight-loss Tracker: A Daily Calorie, Carb, Protein, Fat and Exercise Journal to Help You Lose Weight and Inches* (Apple Press; 2005)

Cooper, Mick and Baker, Peter *The MANual: The Complete Man's Guide to Life* (Thorsons; London, 1996)

Diagram Group, The *Man's Body: An Owner's Manual* (Wordsworth Editions; Ware, Hertfordshire, 1998)

Editors of 'Men's Health' *"Men's Health" Best: Turn Fat into Muscle* (Macmillan; London, 2005)

Egger, Garry *Trim for Life: 201 Tips for Effective Weight Control* (Allen & Unwin; St Leonards, Australia, 1997)

Gauntlett-Gilbert, Jeremy and Grace, Clare *Overcoming Weight Problems* (Robinson Publications; 2005)

Goer, Imah *Shag Yourself Slim* (Crombie Jardine Publishing Limited; 2004)

Goffi, Toni *One Minute Exercise Book* (Help Yourself; 2005)

Gullo, Stephen *The Thin Commandments* (Macmillan; London, 2005)

Inlander, Charles B et al *Men's Health and Wellness Encyclopaedia* (Macmillan; New York, 1998)

Lindberg, Fedon Alexander *The Greek Doctor's Diet: A Simple Delicious Mediterranean Approach to Eating and Exercise Designed to Keep You Naturally Slim and Help You to Avoid Syndrome X, Insulin Resistance, Diabetes and Heart Disease* (Rodale; 2005)

McGraw, Phillip C *The Ultimate Weight Solution Food Guide* (Pocket Books; 2005)

Pollard, Jim *All Right, Mate?* (Orion; 1999)

Ursell, Amanda *What are You Really Eating? How to be Label Savvy* (previously *L is for Labels*) (Hay House; 2005)

Credits

Editor	Ian Barnes
Editorial director	Matthew Minter
Page build	James Robertson
Technical illustrations	Pete Shoemark and Mark Stevens
Photography	Paul Buckland, Penny Cox, Bob Jex, Tracey Robertson and Mark Stevens
Models	Ian Barnes, Richard Head, Bob Jex, Aidan Robertson, Aisling Robertson, James Robertson and Mark Stevens

A range of cycling books is available from Haynes Publishing:

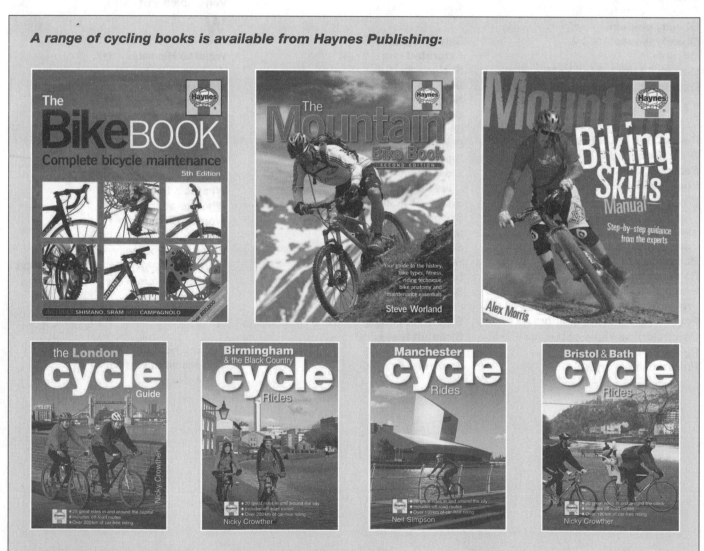

Available from all good bookshops or online at **www.haynes.co.uk**